A BALL IN MY HEAD

The journey of a brain tumour survivor

Janani
Amarasuriya

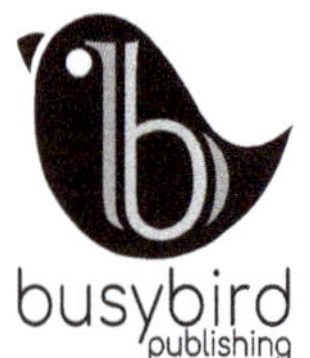

Busybird Publishing
2/118 Para Road
Montmorency, Victoria
Australia 3094
www.busybird.com.au

With heartfelt gratitude, I dedicate this book to
Dr Jun Kim, my exceptional brain surgeon, and
to Dr Cecilia Gzell, my radiation oncologist.
Without their expertise, compassion and
unwavering care, I would not be here today.

I also wish to extend a sincere thank you to my
parents, my sister, Uncle Chandra and all my
other family members for their love and
support throughout this journey.

To my friends: your kindness, prayers, and
moral support have meant everything to me. I
could not have made it through this
without all of you.

Contents

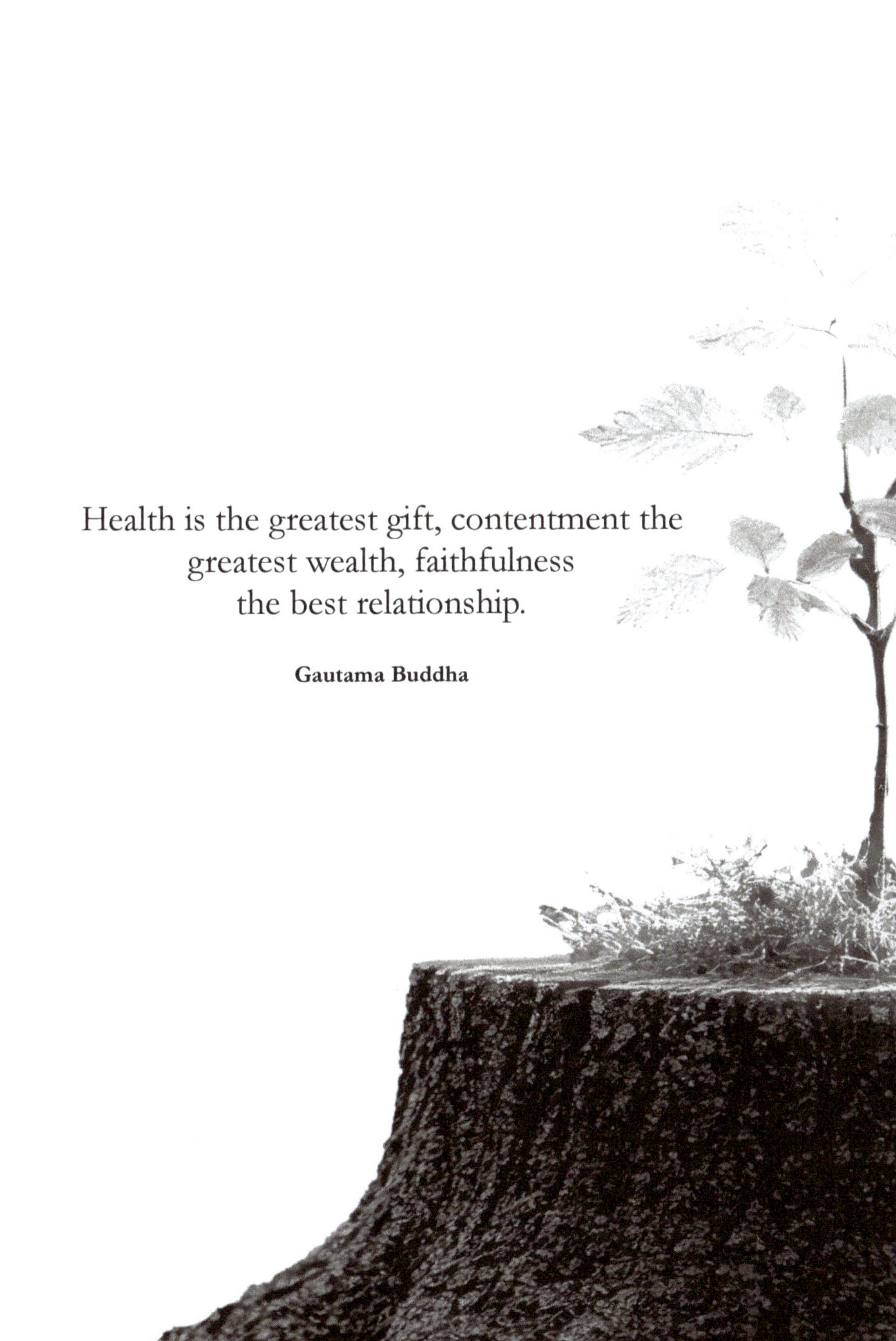

Health is the greatest gift, contentment the
greatest wealth, faithfulness
the best relationship.

Gautama Buddha

Introduction

Before my own ordeal began, I thought trauma belonged to stories of war, loss, or violent crime – events far removed from my daily life. Illness was stressful, of course, but I couldn't fathom how deeply a diagnosis could shake a person to their core. That changed the day I heard the words: 'You have a brain tumour.'

The moment those words reached me, they echoed in the air, impossible to grasp and yet impossible to ignore. My legs felt weak, my heart pounded, and the world tilted slightly off its axis. It was as if my mind had gone numb before my body could register the shock – an icy, heavy feeling settling over everything familiar.

In the hours and days that followed, the news haunted my thoughts, refusing to let go. I remember lying awake at night, staring at the ceiling, replaying the doctor's words and searching for answers that simply weren't there. The uncertainty was suffocating as I wondered what the future held.

The immediate aftermath brought moments when fear threatened to swallow me whole. Everyday routines – having a cuppa in the morning or chatting with my sister – were interrupted by waves of anxiety and disbelief. I found myself watching the sunrise, wondering if I would be able to appreciate such beauty tomorrow, or if everything would soon be different. My cat, Archie, curled up beside me, offering silent comfort through sleepless nights. These small moments of tenderness became anchors when it felt like I was drifting in a sea of uncertainty.

Despite the weight of the diagnosis, I knew I had a choice. I could let despair take over, or I could try to find the light in the darkness. Giving up was never an option. I clung to the 'glass half-full' approach, willing myself to believe that I could muster the strength to fight. It wasn't easy – optimism sometimes felt like a fragile shell – but it helped me face each day, one breath at a time.

Throughout this journey, one lesson has grown clearer than any other: life is a gift, and each new day is a privilege. In the chaos of appointments and treatments, I discovered the meaning behind living in the present – a practice I've tried to follow since childhood as a Buddhist. The future is always uncertain, and all we have for sure is today. I stopped obsessing over trivial worries, choosing instead to focus on what truly mattered. There were mornings when the scent of jasmine outside my window or playing with my cat brought a kind of peace I'd never known before.

I also realised the importance of expressing gratitude and love without delay. There was a moment after my diagnosis when I felt overwhelmed by the support from my parents, my sister, and my friends. In the middle of a sleepless night, I picked up my phone and sent heartfelt messages to those who mattered most. Their replies brought tears to my eyes and reminded me that we shouldn't hold back words of appreciation or affection – life is too short for regrets. These moments deepened my connections, making every conversation and shared memory richer and more meaningful.

As I share my story, I invite you, dear reader, to pause and reflect on your own journey. What words or feelings have you left unspoken? What simple pleasures or relationships have you overlooked in the rush of daily life? If my experience has taught me anything, it's that the true value of our time lies in being present, expressing gratitude, and cherishing the people who walk beside us – today and every day.

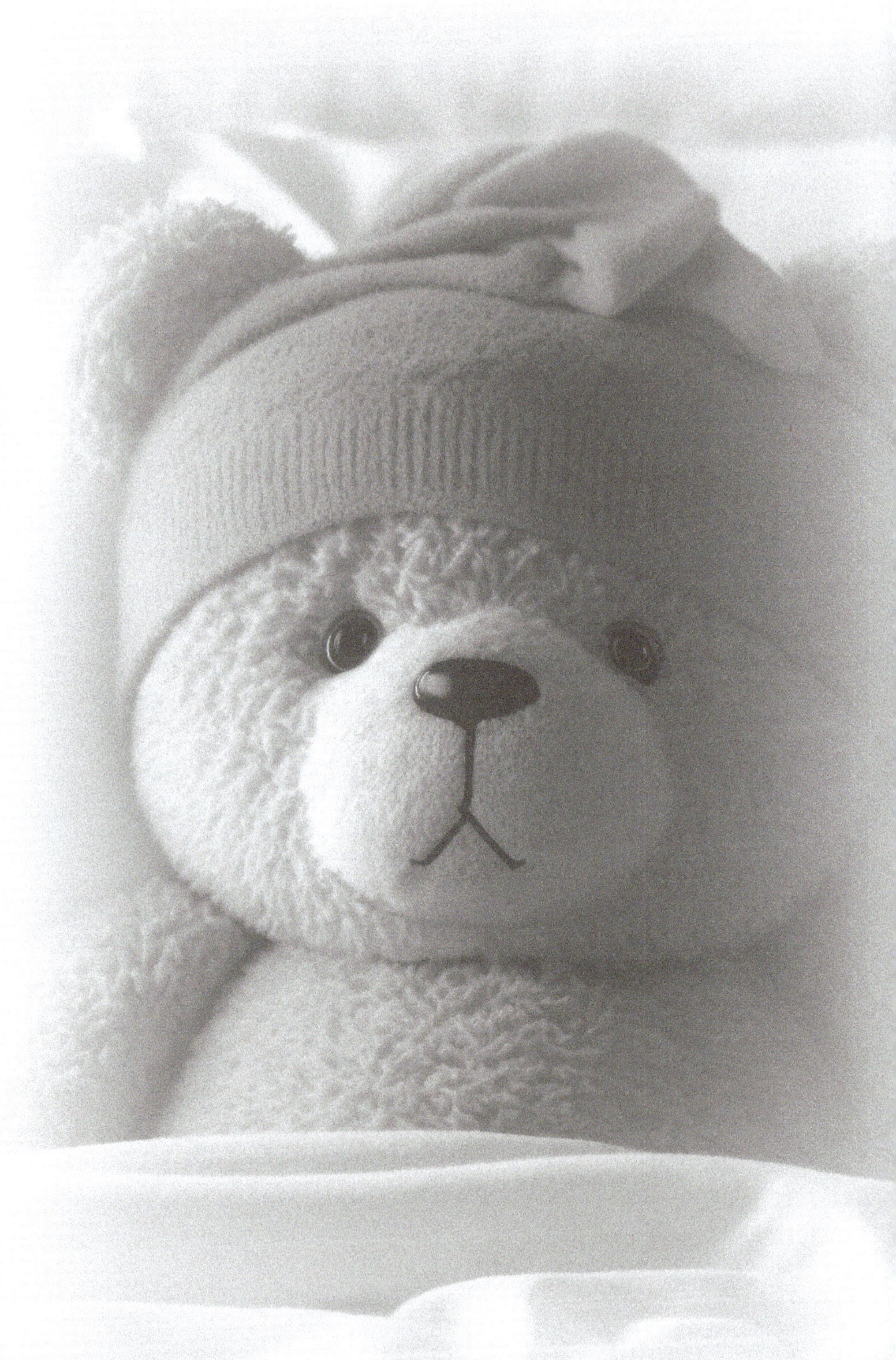

Chapter

1

Numbness and Other Symptoms

It was a chilly morning in June 2023 when I first noticed something was off – my face felt numb on one side. That odd sensation unsettled me. I tried to brush it off, hoping it was just a fluke, but as the days passed, the changes became harder to ignore. My world started losing its flavours and scents; my ability to taste and smell faded, making everything from my morning cuppa to dinner with friends feel disappointingly bland. Night-time was no longer comforting, as my vision grew blurry in the dark. These little changes crept into my daily life, chipping away at my sense of normalcy and leaving me feeling anxious about what might come next.

As winter dragged on, fatigue became my constant companion. One day, I slept through the entire afternoon and evening – a rare occurrence for someone usually up at sunrise. This ongoing exhaustion made even simple tasks feel monumental, and I started to worry that something serious was going on. I confided in my friend Mary, who works as a pharmacist. She suggested some health supplements to boost my energy, and while they helped a bit, that bone-deep tiredness lingered. Headaches soon joined the mix, making days at work and quiet evenings at home harder to enjoy.

Connecting Symptoms and Seeking Help

At first, I tried to convince myself that these problems were just the lingering effects of COVID – I'd had it about a month earlier, and the idea of 'long COVID' seemed plausible. I kept waiting for things to improve, but by September 2023, the symptoms only got worse. By this point, I realised I couldn't keep hoping things would resolve on their own. On 27 September 2023, I decided to book an appointment with my GP, Dr Mark Fitzmaurice, in Hornsby – a date that stands out as a turning point in my journey.

During my visit, Dr Fitzmaurice took my concerns seriously. He ran a thorough check-up, asking questions and testing my reflexes. He examined the numbness on my face. When using a cotton bud to touch the white area of my eyes, he noticed my reflexes were slow in one eye. He explained that, unlike typical post-COVID symptoms which tend to affect both sides equally, my numbness was only on one side – a clue that something else might be going on. Hearing this, I felt a mix of relief and dread, knowing we were getting closer to answers but also fearing what those answers might be.

Understanding that my symptoms needed specialist attention, Dr Fitzmaurice quickly referred me to a neurologist. That afternoon, I found myself at Hornsby Ku-ring-gai Hospital, sitting nervously in Dr Chung's clinic. Dr Chung examined my vision, checked my reflexes, and ran some sensory tests. One test involved tasting foods with different flavours – salty, sweet, bitter, sour – to see if I could still identify them. He also explained what he was ruling out: stroke, Parkinson's disease, Bell's palsy, and other neurological disorders. Each test felt like another step into the unknown, and the uncertainty weighed heavily on me.

Since the cause of my symptoms remained a mystery, Dr Chung recommended an MRI scan. For anyone unfamiliar, an MRI (magnetic resonance imaging) is a special medical test that uses powerful magnets and radio waves to take detailed pictures of the inside of your body – especially the brain. This scan helps doctors see if anything unusual is happening beneath the surface. Within a few days, I had the MRI done. Waiting for the results was nerve-wracking, as I tried to keep myself busy and distracted, but the anxiety never really left.

Looking back, the weeks between June and September 2023 were like moving through a fog – each new symptom and test added layers of uncertainty and worry. Through each appointment and sleepless night, I found myself reflecting on how quickly life can change, and how important it is to listen to your body and seek help when things don't feel right.

Chapter

2

The Day that Changed my Life

I visited my GP to find out my prognosis. I never imagined I would hear the news he gave me that day.

He held the MRI scan and report, visibly worried. To his shock, the results showed a 4 centimetre tumour in my brain near my right trigeminal nerve. Although he explained these types of growths are usually benign tumours, he still seemed worried.

Dr Fitzmaurice has been my GP for several years; he is a compassionate doctor who genuinely cares for his patients. He was particularly concerned because I was only 53 years old. Without delay, he referred me to neurosurgeon Dr Brian Owler and asked me to go straight to the Sydney Adventist Hospital (San Hospital) in Wahroonga, to see Dr Owler at the emergency department that same day.

Referral to the Neurosurgeon

I was shocked to be diagnosed with a brain tumour. I promptly called Dr Brian Owler's office to arrange an urgent consultation. The receptionist answered and explained that Dr Owler was currently on a flight to the USA for a holiday. She reassured me that during his absence, his associate, Dr Yun Kim, would be caring for all his patients. She also mentioned that Dr Kim was presently at the hospital, making his rounds after having performed surgery on his patients earlier that day.

I had already learned that Dr Owler is regarded as one of the best neurosurgeons in Australia – if not the very best. This gave me confidence that he would only entrust his patients to someone of equal calibre. I decided to go directly to the hospital and wait for Dr Kim, trusting that I would be in highly capable hands during this critical time.

On my day off from work, I opted to take the train to my GP appointment due to fatigue and not feeling comfortable driving. Shortly thereafter, my ex- husband Ravin, who remains a close friend, contacted me. Upon hearing of the situation, he offered to pick me up and drive me to the hospital, as he was working from home. I sincerely appreciated his support during this time.

As I waited for my ride, the reality hit me hard, and fear set in. Tears streamed down my face as I sat outside, struggling to believe what was happening. I know I am not perfect, but I have never intentionally hurt anyone. Life felt so unfair, and I wondered if it was past karma from a previous existence. As a Buddhist, that explanation made sense to me.

I then called my boyfriend Brian and shared the news. Brian's voice trembled with worry, but he gently reminded me to stay positive until we heard from the surgeon. His reassurance helped steady my nerves, even though I knew he wished he could be there. I assured Brian that I would update him as soon as I spoke to the surgeon, knowing he couldn't leave work at short notice but wanting to keep him in the loop.

My thoughts went to the journey of a close friend who had faced a far more daunting diagnosis – stage 4 lung cancer that had metastasised to her brain. She endured multiple surgeries, followed by rounds of chemotherapy and radiotherapy, yet through sheer determination and perseverance, she managed to overcome her illness. Witnessing her strength and resilience gave me hope during my own difficult time. Motivated by her example, I decided to trust my doctors and take proactive steps to address my situation, believing that a positive attitude and decisive action would help me navigate the challenges ahead.

Emergency Department Admission and Meeting with the Neurosurgeon

Upon arrival at the hospital emergency department, I waited anxiously to be called in. My thoughts kept drifting to Archie, my cat, who was alone at home. I worried that he must be feeling anxious and missing me.

After waiting for approximately six hours, I was finally seen by the registrar. She conducted a preliminary check, asked me some routine questions, and then brought me into a room within the patient waiting area. She instructed a nurse to ensure I was comfortable and provided me with something to eat and drink, as she anticipated my wait would be lengthy.

The area included a bed, a television and a chair, which allowed me to rest. I ate a little, then phoned Ravin to update him, explaining that I would be seeing the surgeon in a few hours and, since it was getting late, asking him to check on Archie for me. Ravin reassured me that he would pick me up when I was ready to go home. I felt relieved and grateful for his continued friendship, and for the fact that he lived close to the hospital.

Eventually, I met Dr Yun Kim, who explained my diagnosis in detail. He informed me that I had a grade 1 meningioma, which is generally a benign tumour. However, he noted that due to its considerable size and its position near the trigeminal nerve, surgery to remove the tumour was necessary. Dr Kim warned that if left untreated, the tumour could grow larger and potentially cause serious complications such as seizures or stroke within a couple of years. He also explained that delaying surgery further could increase risks associated with age, including developing dementia, which might result in me becoming ineligible for surgery in the future. He was candid, stating that if I were a member of his own family, he would strongly recommend proceeding with surgery, as it was the only option for a tumour of this size. He also emphasised that this would be the most significant operation I had ever experienced.

I asked Dr Kim about the expected recovery period. He recommended at least two months off work and three months without driving after surgery. When I inquired about the risks, he told me there was a two percent chance of stroke. Dr Kim also introduced me to his assistant surgeon, Dr Roshni, and scheduled my surgery for two weeks' time.

With my immediate family living in Perth and me alone in Sydney, I asked the doctors whether it would be possible to have the surgery closer to my parents. However, the consensus was that Sydney offered better medical options for my condition. Dr Kim expressed concern about my circumstances, stressing how vital family support would be during recovery. He offered to talk to my family about what to expect during recovery.

Discussions with Family and Friends

After returning home from the hospital, I found myself enveloped in a wave of fear and sadness. The reality of my diagnosis set in with a heaviness that made it hard to breathe, and the uncertainty of what lay ahead took hold of my thoughts. Alone in my apartment, every sound felt amplified – my mind raced as I tried to make sense of what this would mean for my future. The solitude was confronting, but in that quiet moment, I realised how much I needed my loved ones to anchor me.

My first instinct was to reach out to my parents and my sister Udani, needing to share the burden of the news. The conversation was emotional; hearing their shock and concern brought the gravity of the situation into sharper focus. They immediately wanted to fly to Sydney to be by my side, but I reassured them that their support would be most needed during my recovery after surgery. This realisation – that they would drop everything for me – reminded me of the strength and unconditional love that family offers, especially in times of crisis. I made a conscious effort to ease their worries, telling them about the wonderful group of friends I have in Sydney whom would help me through the initial weeks.

When my sister offered to come and stay, I felt a mix of gratitude and concern. I knew how much I needed her, but the thought of her leaving my niece and nephew unsettled me; her children are still young, and their lives would be disrupted. After some reflection, I asked her to remain at home for now, feeling it was best not to add further upheaval to our family. This decision, although difficult, taught me that accepting help sometimes means considering what's best for everyone involved.

Seeking clarity, I sent my scans and medical reports to several family members who are medical professionals. The transition from fear to action gave me a small sense of control. My scans were reviewed by Saman (a practicising GP, and the husband of one of my cousins in Brisbane), Uncle Sarath in England (a retired ENT surgeon), Aunt Hema in England (a retired GP), and Uncle Chandra in

Germany (a retired senior nurse). They unanimously advised me to proceed with surgery. Their calm expertise steadied my nerves, and knowing they had my best interests at heart gave me the confidence to move forward. With their guidance, I booked my operation for 11 October 2023 at the Seventh Day Adventist Hospital.

Brian, my boyfriend at the time, was an invaluable support during this uncertain time. Together, we dug deep into researching Dr Kim, determined to ensure I was entrusting my health to an experienced and reputable surgeon. We scoured hospital websites for profiles and credentials, checked the Australian Health Practitioner Regulation Agency (AHPRA) for his medical registration, and searched for patient reviews on health forums and Google. We even looked up hospital ratings and any articles that mentioned Dr Kim's outcomes or reputation. Each positive review and credential gave me a little more confidence, slowly easing my nerves about the upcoming surgery.

When it came to understanding the two percent stroke risk, Brian and I pored over clinical studies and reputable medical websites like the Mayo Clinic, wanting to grasp what those numbers truly meant. We discussed the statistics at length, weighing the risks against the benefits. The knowledge that the risk, while significant, was relatively low in the context of such a major operation helped somewhat, but I couldn't help feeling a wave of anxiety each time I thought about it. Brian's background as a fellow regulatory scientist (more senior to me), coupled with his bio-chemistry knowledge and medical know-how, was incredibly reassuring — he broke down the information for me in a calm and rational way, helping me see that the odds were in my favour. In those moments, I felt deeply grateful to have Brian by my side, guiding me through the uncertainty and reminding me that I wasn't facing these decisions alone.

It was in that moment, as the date was set, that a new resolve started to take shape. I wasn't alone in making this decision – I was surrounded by a safety net of experience and love.

The following day, I called my cousins in Brisbane and Melbourne, as well as a handful of close friends. Sharing the daunting news felt surreal. I tried my best to sound calm and reassuring, not wanting to alarm anyone; beneath my composed tone, the terror of the unknown lingered. As the conversations unfolded, I was deeply moved by their immediate concern and their assurances to support me in any way I needed. Each gesture – whether a comforting word, a promise to visit, or simply listening – helped chip away at my isolation, replacing it with warmth and communal strength.

Another layer of reassurance came when Saman recognised the difficulties associated with the tumour's size and position, yet confirmed that surgery was the most appropriate course of action. This candid conversation, delivered with compassion and clarity, helped me trust the path I was on. Later, Prasanna – married to my cousin Wayomee – shared that his mum had undergone surgery for a benign brain tumour years ago in Sri Lanka and went on to live many long years. Hearing about Prasanna's mum was incredibly comforting; her story offered hope and a reminder that advances in medical care, combined with courageous decisions, could lead to positive outcomes. I held onto this hope, allowing it to soften the fear and inspire a more optimistic outlook. The knowledge that I'd be having my surgery in Australia, where new techniques are available, further buoyed my spirits.

As the date drew nearer, my friend Anushka said she would come to Sydney a few days before the surgery to help with the last-minute arrangements – a simple gesture that meant more than words could express. She, too, shared a story: one of her close family friends had recently had a benign brain tumour removed in Sydney and recovered well with time. Hearing about this recent success made the challenge ahead seem less daunting, and the reassurance in Anushka's voice gave me the courage to face what was coming.

Reflecting on these moments, I am struck by how each conversation, each gesture – no matter how small – wove together a tapestry of comfort and connection. Whether it was family members offering unwavering support from afar, friends showing up in person, or stories of hope shared over phone calls, I found myself slowly letting go of the sense of loneliness. The journey ahead was still daunting, but knowing I had such a strong support network made all the difference. Their empathy and encouragement didn't just help me cope; they transformed my mindset, filling me with gratitude and giving me the strength to approach surgery – and recovery – with hope and resilience.

After confirming my surgery date with the Sydney Adventist Hospital, a nervous anticipation settled in – as if the reality of what lay ahead had finally landed. One of my first priorities was making sure Archie, my beloved cat, would be safe and cared for. Since my operation would require several weeks of recovery, I wanted Archie to be somewhere familiar and safe.

I organised for him to be boarded at his usual cattery, Puss 'n' Boots in Dural, which is operated by Archie's vet Katie and her husband Michael, starting on the day of my operation. They always took great care of Archie every time I left him there, so that put me at ease. Archie always seemed happy and relaxed when I picked him up, often purring loudly as soon as he saw me, which reassured me that he was comfortable and well cared for in my absence. The staff were understanding about the uncertainty of my hospital stay and kindly agreed to keep Archie for as long as needed, which eased one of my biggest worries. With practical matters like Archie's care settled, I turned my attention to ensuring my legal affairs were in order.

A few days before my surgery, my sister came to Sydney. My oldest friend in Australia, Celine, also visited from Perth for the weekend. Celine has always felt like another sister to me. We first met as teenagers at a Sri Lankan New Year festival in Perth back in 1988. She was so close to my family that she even lived with us during her final year of college – her school was nearer to our house. My parents cared for her as if she was their third daughter, and my sister treated her like another older sister. The three of us have always shared a special bond.

Having my sister and Celine with me lifted my spirits. Their company brought comfort and a much-needed distraction from my worries. One day, we drove to Milsons Point and wandered around the city. The air was crisp and salty, and the Harbour Bridge glimmered under the afternoon sun. I felt a mixture of nerves and hope as we walked along the footpath, chatting and laughing. The familiar sound of ferries and the distant hum of the city made me appreciate being surrounded by people who cared for me.

We met Eisha at a café in Crows Nest. Eisha used to be our neighbour in Perth. She's also a close childhood friend of my sister and a longstanding family friend. The café was cosy, with the aroma of fresh coffee and baked goods filling the air. We settled into a sunlit corner and caught up on life. Eisha, warm and thoughtful, asked about my health. Her concern was so genuine it brought a lump to my throat. She assured me that I could reach out for help at any time. My sister seemed relieved knowing that Eisha – one of her closest friends – lived nearby in Sydney. It gave her extra peace of mind, knowing I had another caring person in my corner.

On Sunday, just before my surgery, my sister and Celine prepared to head home. That same day, Prasanna happened to be in Sydney on business. He dropped by with a container of Sri Lankan food that my cousin, his wife Wayomee, had lovingly prepared and sent. The moment I opened the lid, the kitchen filled with the scent of spicy curries and coconut. We warmed the food for lunch – rich flavours, familiar and comforting. I thanked Prasanna and asked him to pass on my gratitude to Wayomee. Sharing that meal was more than just nourishment; it was a reminder of family and tradition, and it made me feel cared for.

Prasanna offered to drive my sister and Celine to the airport. I was grateful for his help. We hugged, exchanged goodbyes, and wished each other well. Watching them leave, I felt a wave of sadness but also deep gratitude. These visits reminded me that I wasn't facing my challenges alone.

Looking back, I realise how much these relationships have helped me in tough times – not just now but in the past, too. My family and friends have always shown up when I needed them most. Their kindness has taught me the power of community, and it's something I hope to pass on. I want to be there for others when they face uncertainty or hardship, just as my loved ones have been there for me. In moments like these, it's clear that support and connection are what truly carry us through.

That same day, a few close friends from my gym and Zumba classes came for afternoon tea at my place. They included Ariel, Vivian, Magda, Michael, Jeet, Carmela and one of our Zumba gym instructors named Alfonso. Sharing the news of my upcoming surgery with them was daunting, but their concern and reassurance were a source of comfort. I refrained from sharing too many details, wanting to keep the mood light, but when I mentioned it was brain surgery, some of them, like Vivian (a retired hospital social worker) and Carmela (an anaesthetic nurse), understood the gravity of the situation. Their understanding and calm presence helped steady my nerves.

Some of my former colleagues from Reckitt Benckiser expressed interest in visiting the day before hospital admission, but I declined, choosing instead to focus on preparing myself mentally and physically.

Throughout all these preparations, the collective support and kindness shown by those around me bolstered my spirits and gave me the strength needed to face what was ahead.

My cousin Sewandi also visited and brought more food to stock in my freezer. She reassured me that when my parents came to Sydney, she'd be there to help if needed. This eased my concerns about them being alone at a challenging time. We agreed to discuss the best plan for my parents by phone in the coming days. Sewandi, one of my father's nieces, has always been a kind and caring person. I knew my parents would be in good hands with her, especially since she's married to a doctor and has a sensible, level-headed approach. I've always felt lucky to have such a wonderful family.

Preparing for Surgery

Preparing for surgery meant tackling all the necessary paperwork and arrangements. I reviewed and updated my will, making sure it accurately reflected my wishes. Additionally, I appointed my sister as my power of attorney, granting her the authority to manage my affairs should the need arise. Throughout this process, I was fortunate to have my close friend Joan, who is also my lawyer, by my side. Her guidance and support helped me navigate the legal requirements, and having her expertise gave me peace of mind that everything was sorted. As I ticked off each item on my checklist, I felt a sense of control returning, even as uncertainty lingered.

I also made sure to discuss Archie's future care with my sister, knowing just how much she loves him too. To make things concrete, I set aside funds for Archie's ongoing expenses and formally appointed my sister, my cousin Lalanthi and our friend Eisha (who all love cats) as his guardians in my will, ensuring they would have everything they needed to look after him. Taking these steps gave me peace of mind, knowing Archie would always be loved and safe, no matter what happened.

As I navigated these arrangements, the support from friends and family became increasingly important. I kept my cousins and friends updated with regular messages, so everyone was aware of my progress and plans. Their encouragement and steady presence made the daunting process feel much less isolating.

I also appointed different friends and family members for various tasks. My sister was to update the family members and friends, Brian to update my colleagues and some friends he knew, and Ravin to update our mutual friends.

We decided my parents should fly to Brisbane and stay with Sewandi and Saman on the day of my surgery. If any complications arose, they could quickly fly to

Sydney; otherwise, they would come after my surgery was completed. I knew that seeing me in a vulnerable state would be stressful for them, so I wanted to spare them that anxiety by ensuring they were surrounded by supportive family. Having Saman there was especially reassuring – his medical expertise gave me confidence that my parents would be cared for, no matter what happened. Knowing that practical arrangements and family support were in place helped me feel more at ease about their wellbeing during such a challenging time.

I was grateful for my extended family, with several cousins in Brisbane and Melbourne who could offer support. Still, I realised the recovery would be lengthy, and it would be unreasonable to expect my ageing parents, sister, or cousins with their own families to provide long-term care. As a result, I asked my uncle Chandra in Germany, a retired nurse and my mother's youngest brother, if he could come to Sydney to help me during my recovery. He lives alone, is in good health, and has always been close to my family. He said of course. His willingness to drop everything for me brought a wave of relief and gratitude, reminding me that I wasn't facing this challenge alone. Uncle Chandra has always been the angel of our family, caring for any relatives or friends in need, and we are all incredibly fortunate to have him.

Anushka arrived two days prior to hospital admission. We went to the local Westfield and bought a few pairs of Peter Alexander pyjama suits for the hospital, as they can be worn as casual loungewear.

I also got my facial hair removed. To her amusement, I explained to Anushka that I wanted to look presentable for the hospital staff.

I even went on a walk with Anushka (to her surprise, as I still had mental strength to do that). Then Anushka helped me to pack a bag; we included the clothes we bought, some toiletries, my medicines and paperwork from the hospital.

Now I was all ready to admit to the hospital the next day.

Hospital Admission

The day before my surgery arrived, bringing with it a quiet sense of inevitability and the need to set everything in order. That morning, Vivian pulled up in her car outside my place – a comforting presence, as she'd offered to help take Archie to the cattery. Vivian, one of my closest gym friends, lives just a few suburbs away and shares my deep affection for animals, especially cats. Her warmth and gentle manner made her the perfect companion for such a bittersweet errand.

With Anushka joining us, the three of us gently coaxed Archie into his carrier, his golden eyes watching me with a mix of trust and confusion. The drive to the cattery was quiet, punctuated by Vivian's soft reassurances to Archie and Anushka's comforting grip on my shoulder.

When we arrived, the ambient sounds of other cats mewing and the subtle antiseptic tang in the air made the reality sink in. As I handed Archie over, a lump formed in my throat – I stroked his soft fur one last time, feeling the familiar warmth beneath my palm and whispering promises that I'd be back for him soon. The uncertainty of how long he would stay there gnawed at me, and I found it hard to let go; Archie is more than a pet – he's family, my little shadow in every room.

Afterwards, wanting to reclaim a sense of normalcy, I took Vivian and Anushka out to brunch in Wahroonga. The café was bright and bustling, the aroma of fresh coffee mingling with the chatter of mornings. As a small gesture of gratitude for their kindness and support, I gave Vivian a pair of delicate cat-shaped earrings – her eyes lit up when she saw them. For Anushka, I chose orchid-shaped earrings; she laughed in surprise, giving me a tight hug. Their genuine delight and the easy laughter we shared helped lighten the weight of the day, reminding me just how lucky I am to be surrounded by such caring friends. In that moment, despite the looming uncertainty, I felt deeply grateful for the strength their companionship gave me.

My good friend Ranadeva, whom I have known since I was eighteen, offered to drive me to the hospital for my surgery. However, since my friend Anushka was already with me and familiar with this part of Sydney from her previous years here, she offered to drop me off using my car. My ex-husband Ravin also offered to drive me. Ranadeva assured me that he was available as a backup in case I needed help with transport, and I appreciated his support. Having friends like Ranadeva, Anushka and Ravin by my side during such a challenging time brought me a deep sense of comfort and reassurance, reminding me how fortunate I am to have such caring people in my life.

In the end, Ravin took Anushka and me to the hospital in his car and went back to his home, as he was working from home. He assured me that he would assist Anushka to get to the airport afterwards.

Brian had to go on a business trip to the Philippines that he couldn't avoid. As a senior manager at his company, his presence was essential. He was unhappy about leaving, especially with my surgery approaching. I could see the worry etched on his face, and I tried to reassure him with a smile, even though I felt anxious inside. I told him it was alright – he had no other choice, and I would be supported by my friends in Sydney and family who were on standby. We said our goodbyes the day before, as he had to fly out that day. Although he was upset to leave, we both understood the necessity of his trip, and I appreciated the support network that would be there for me in his absence.

I was then admitted to the hospital. Although my personal faith is Buddhism, I found comfort in knowing that the hospital is a religious one. As someone with a spiritual outlook on life, this setting provided me with reassurance and peace of mind. I felt confident that I was in capable and caring hands, which eased my anxieties.

As I entered the hospital, a subtle blend of antiseptic and fresh linen filled the air, mingling with the low hum of distant voices and the soft squeak of nurses' shoes in the corridor. The fluorescent lights overhead cast a gentle glow, illuminating the pale walls and polished floors that seemed to stretch endlessly ahead. Anushka carried my hospital bag. I felt a shiver of anticipation mixed with a muted anxiety that sat low in my chest. Anushka was by my side, her presence grounding me as we navigated the winding halls towards the MRI suite.

We were greeted by a nurse who took me into a room, told me to change to a hospital gown and inserted a cannula into my hand so that the technician could inject the contrast fluid during the MRI process. Then I sat in the MRI suite with Anushka. She still had my bag next to her. There was a windowpane with a glass print of beautiful green leaves where we were sitting. I told Anushka they reminded me of Bodhi leaves.

After a few minutes I was called in to the MRI room. Inside the dimly lit room, cold air pressed against my skin, and the metallic tang of the equipment seemed sharper, mingling with the faint scent of hospital disinfectant. I'd had MRIs done before in that same room, so I knew the procedure. The technician was very kind, giving me earplugs and helping me to lay down on the sliding table. As I gazed upwards, I noticed a cross mounted on the ceiling above me. It stood out, carved into the ceiling yet somehow radiant against the white backdrop. The sight of the cross stirred something deep within me; it was as if the walls fell away and I was cradled in a moment of stillness and solace. I was moved into the machine, which felt like a tunnel from a sci-fi film. The ear plugs blocked the loud metallic noise produced by the machine – I also had a button to press if I needed to talk to her during the process if I felt uncomfortable.

My thoughts drifted to my late cousin Layan, whose memory has always been entwined with gentle reassurance. In that suspended moment, I imagined Layan as my guardian angel, watching over me from somewhere just out of sight. When I later told Anushka about the cross, she smiled softly, suggesting perhaps Layan really was with me, offering silent protection from above. The idea soothed me; warmth spread through my chest, replacing fear with a deep, quiet comfort.

Inside the MRI, the world narrowed to sensation and sound. The coldness of the table pressed against my back, seeping through the thin hospital gown and raising goosebumps along my skin. Even through the earplugs, the rhythmic thumping and whirring of the machine reverberated through my body – a metallic heartbeat that filled the dim room and made the air feel thick, almost electric. The sharp, unmistakable scent of disinfectant lingered, mingling with the sterile chill that settled into my bones.

Each pulse of the machine seemed to echo the anxious flutter of my heart. In those tense moments, my thoughts drifted to my parents, my sister, and my friends – each one a vital thread in the tapestry of my life. I could picture them in their separate corners of the world, sending out prayers and hope, their love reaching for me across the sterile boundaries of this room. That love felt tangible, like a comforting blanket wrapped around my trembling form, holding back the tide of anxiety and uncertainty.

I imagined Anushka, waiting just outside, her silent prayer mingling with mine, infusing the antiseptic air with a thread of warmth and faith. Vulnerability settled heavily on me, but it was softened by the realisation that I was not alone; I was buoyed by the care and concern of so many.

When the technician Daniel's calm voice filtered through the microphone, guiding me step by step, I clung to his words as an anchor in this foreign, humming tunnel. Wanting to steady myself – both for the scan and the emotions swirling beneath the surface – I chose to meditate. Closing my eyes, I gathered the love sent from afar, letting it root me firmly in the present moment. My breath became my focus, the in-and-out rhythm offering a counterpoint to the mechanical thump around me. Meditation was a familiar refuge, but in that moment, it became more: a conscious act of gratitude, a way to transform fear into a quiet, inner resilience.

As the scan continued, I noticed the vulnerability that had once made me feel so small had shifted, replaced by a sense of strength I didn't know I possessed. The prayers and hopes of those who cared for me weren't just comforting – they became the scaffolding that held me up. Lying there, surrounded by cold metal and humming machinery, I understood with piercing clarity how deeply I was supported. Gratitude bloomed in my chest, gentle but powerful, reshaping the way I saw both myself and the people who loved me. I emerged from that scan not just examined but fortified – held by the invisible bonds of care, and quietly certain that their strength had become my own.

After the MRI, I was wheeled into another room, the scent of hand sanitiser lingering as Anushka joined me again, phone in hand to capture a few snapshots – her way of lightening the mood with gentle humour. The arrival of my surgeon, Dr Kim, and the assistant surgeon, Dr Roshni, brought a wave of reassurance. Their calm, professional demeanour and warm smiles eased some of the tension knotting my muscles. I introduced them to Anushka, and she snapped a photo of the three of us, capturing a fleeting moment of connection amid the clinical setting. Their presence – steady and kind – reminded me that I was in skilled hands. I remember my aunt in England saying to pray for the medical team too, so that they get the strength to carry out a successful surgery. I silently said a prayer for them.

Then, with a gentle knock and a soft-spoken greeting, a wardsman arrived to escort me to the surgical theatre. Soon after, it was time for Anushka and me to part. There was a heavy stillness in the air as she gathered my valuables and tucked them away safely. We hugged tightly, her arms enveloping me in a final cocoon of strength and affection. Her whispered well-wishes lingered in my ears even after she had left, the echo of her support carrying me into the next stage of the journey.

As I was wheeled down the corridor, the cool hospital air prickled my skin, and the quiet, methodical movements of the hospital staff offered reassurance. The world narrowed to the rolling rhythm of the trolley, the muted lights overhead, and the faint scent of eucalyptus from a passing nurse's hand cream. As the doors to the theatre swung open, I took a final breath, carrying with me the warmth of my loved ones' prayers and the memory of the cross – a quiet beacon in a moment of uncertainty.

Left briefly alone, I sat in silence, heart thudding, senses heightened to every tick of the clock and muffled sound in the hallway. I reflected on the tapestry of relationships that sustained me – friends and family whose prayers, presence, and unwavering love were woven around me like a soft, protective shawl. Their support did not erase my fear, but it rendered it smaller, manageable – something I could face with courage.

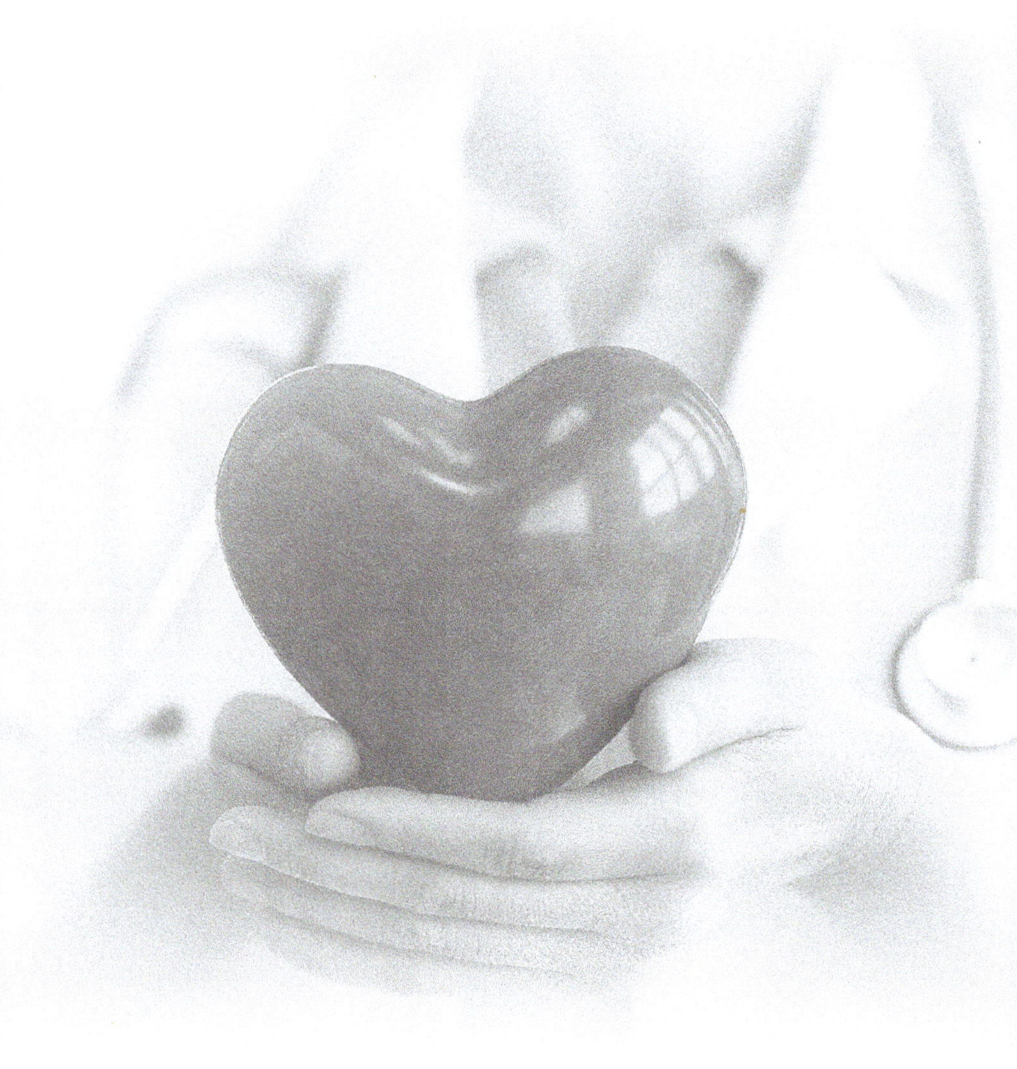

Chapter

3

The Surgery and the First Few Days

After I was taken into the operating theatre area by the wardsman, I recall the anaesthetist speaking with me about general anaesthesia. They were standard medical questions – whether I have any chronic conditions like hypertension, what medications I am currently taking, and when I last ate or drank anything. Following this, I was administered a sedative and anaesthetic.

After that, my memory goes blank; I only remember waking up later in the neurology ward surrounded by nurses. I had no sense of how much time had passed – it felt as if I had been absent from the world.

When I finally woke up, my mind was foggy and my body felt unfamiliar, heavy with exhaustion and the lingering effects of anaesthesia. The faces around me were blurred at first, but gradually I could make out Anushka and Ravin by my bedside, their anxious eyes searching mine for any sign of recognition. I later learned from my surgeon that the operation had lasted twelve hours – yet thankfully, it had been successful. He told me I'd spent three days in intensive care, and there had been real concern when I didn't regain consciousness for a long time. Hearing this, I felt a strange mix of gratitude and vulnerability – my life had hung in the balance, and I had been completely unaware.

Anushka told me she'd seen the surgeon straight after the surgery; she said he looked utterly exhausted, his shoulders slumped from the weight of such a complex procedure.

The surgeon gently moved my left hand, testing for any response, and Anushka instinctively began lifting my hand as well. Her hands were steady, but her voice was soft and trembling with hope. A nurse nearby noticed Anushka's actions and, impressed by her instincts, asked if she had nursing experience. Anushka explained her experience with her father's recovery from a stroke, and the nurse offered a nod of understanding, her tone kind and approving. That small exchange was a reminder of how care sometimes comes from unexpected places, and how much the people in my life wanted to help in any way they could.

I was then moved to a room in the neurology ward. My parents arrived not long afterwards with Uncle Lucky and Aunty Anoja, our long-term family friends. Relief washed over my mother's face when I recognised her and my father.

I remember murmuring 'Ammi (Mum) and Thathi (Dad) – you are here.' Everyone was also relieved when I could answer the surgeon's questions – my name, where I was, and what day it was. The surgeon seemed pleased with my responses.

Aunty Anoja, who used to be a doctor in Sri Lanka, also asked me how I was and she looked relieved when I mumbled I felt alright. Uncle Lucky also said hello with a very concerned look in his eyes. It must have been a shock for them to see me in such a state, when they'd known me since I was about six years old.

In that moment, I appreciated the strength of my relationships, and the silent teamwork that was gently stitching me back together, one small step at a time. I realised just how much my wellbeing meant to my parents, and how much I cherished their presence. The warmth of their support lingered with me as I was moved to the neurology ward, a comforting reminder that I was never truly alone on this journey.

The nurses in the neurology ward at the Sydney Adventist Hospital were truly exceptional. They showed unwavering kindness and attention, making sure I felt cared for during every moment of my stay. My surgeon visited me every day, patiently checking on my progress and keeping my family informed. He even took the time to call my sister Udani, who lived all the way in Perth, so she could stay up to date with my recovery.

The chief speech pathologist was responsible for determining what I should eat or drink. She first told me I could only have thick liquids. I always felt thirsty but was not allowed to have thin liquids like water, so I remember drinking a lot of the thick liquid they provided. It didn't taste nice but it was tolerable. After a few days, I was allowed food and water, to my delight. Later I was told they couldn't allow me thin liquids or food at first due to the risk of choking, as my lungs were not yet at full capacity.

Dr Roshni, the assistant surgeon, was a young Indian doctor whose compassion left a deep impression on me. She visited regularly, not just to monitor my condition, but also to look after my parents. I'll never forget the nights she stayed with me until midnight, quietly offering comfort and reassurance. Her dedication and warmth made a difficult time that much more bearable.

Every day, physiotherapists came to help me regain my strength. In the beginning, I couldn't even sit up in bed on my own. Their encouragement was constant, and when I finally managed to sit upright, there was a ripple of celebration. The chief physiotherapist was so moved by my progress that she hugged my mother, sharing in our relief and happiness. The support from the entire medical team made me feel incredibly lucky, even amid my struggles.

Despite these milestones, my body remained weak. Sitting up was a huge effort, and I still couldn't sit straight, speak clearly, walk, or stand without support. I remember one day the nurses saying a small neck cushion would help, so my parents and Ravin went to look for one. I also remember feeling very uncomfortable as the urinary catheter was still attached to me. Nurses were popping up frequently to take blood pressure measurements and to ensure I was passing urine. They performed CT scans of my bladder and bowels to check that my body was functioning properly. Exhaustion was my constant companion.

Throughout it all, my parents visited every day, as did Brian and Ravin. Other loved ones came often, their presence forming a circle of support around me. One moment stands out: Brian and Ravin shook hands in my hospital room – a gesture that carried real weight, as they had never been in the same room together before. That simple act of respect and acknowledgment meant more to me than words could express, showing that even old boundaries could soften in the face of shared care.

At night, the television above my bed would flicker with news from around the world. One evening I watched, in horror, as a war unfolded in Gaza. The scenes were devastating: hospitals destroyed, children and families caught in violence and pain. It was a jarring contrast to the safety and comfort I received in my own hospital room. Watching the suffering of others, I felt a deep ache of empathy and helplessness. It made me acutely aware of my own good fortune – to be in a peaceful country, receiving world-class medical care. Each night before I drifted to sleep, I said a prayer for those families in Gaza. My own struggle felt smaller compared to the unimaginable hardship they faced. The images haunted me, reminding me of the fragility of life and the privilege of safety. My gratitude ran deeper for the sanctuary I found in the hospital and the people who cared for me.

During my recovery, I received many flower deliveries from friends and colleagues. My gym friends – Magda, Viv and Kaveri – brought beautiful bouquets. Other friends, including Rana, Viktoria, Siva, Frank, Ronaldo, Joan and colleagues from Roche, also reached out with flowers and messages of encouragement. The nurses often commented on how lovely the flowers looked, brightening both my room and my spirits. Each gift was a reminder that I was surrounded by love and support, even when I felt most vulnerable.

Chapter

4

Recovery at the Sydney Adventist Hospital

Approximately one week following my surgery, I celebrated my 54th birthday while still recovering at the Sydney Adventist Hospital. The nurses went out of their way to lift my spirits by decorating my area with balloons. My priest, Ajahn Sujato, visited alongside meditation group friends Depika and Radha. Ajahn Sujato offered a blessing and led a brief meditation session. During this time, I found myself unable to sit up properly or bow to the priest, as my body and hands remained in shock from the operation.

My parents marked the occasion by ordering a birthday cake, which they shared with the nurses and doctors caring for me. Throughout this experience, I felt immense gratitude for my surgeon and the entire medical team, recognising that I might not have had another birthday to celebrate without their dedication and expertise.

Throughout my recovery at the Sydney Adventist Hospital, visitors played a vital role in lifting my spirits and reminding me of the care surrounding me. Their presence, and the tokens they left behind, filled my hospital room with warmth and life, even when I drifted in and out of sleep. Sometimes, I'd awaken to the gentle scent of flowers and spot handwritten cards, evidence of thoughtful friends who'd come while I was resting. Each bouquet and message offered comfort, letting me know I was never truly alone.

My gym friends, Vivian and Magda had visited together one afternoon. I was resting, so I was unaware of their visit. I later learned from Vivian that Magda, deeply shaken by seeing me so frail, had begun crying in the lift after their visit. The genuine emotion showed just how much my wellbeing mattered to them. The vibrant colours and subtle fragrance of their flowers lingered after they left, a gentle reminder of their love and concern.

On another occasion, Ariel – another close friend from the gym – and one of our Zumba instructors arrived on Halloween, on their way to a Halloween themed class. They were dressed as skeletons, their costumes adding a playful energy to the ward. The nurses found their visit amusing and uplifting. Despite the gravity of my situation, their cheerful presence brought moments of levity; I later heard that Ariel, too, was overcome with sadness and cried in the lift after seeing me so unwell. Kaveri visited one day while I was resting and was visibly shocked by what she saw. When

I woke up, I found she'd left a birthday gift and flowers. Heidi, Lavinia and Birgit, my former colleagues and now friends, visited briefly; they seemed shocked, and later I heard Heidi also cried in the lift.

Later that week, Vivian returned on her own. By then, I was feeling a little stronger, and Brian happened to be visiting as well. With the hospital staff's permission, they wheeled me outside so I could enjoy some fresh air and sunlight. The spring day was glorious – the birdsong mingled with the rustling leaves, and the gentle warmth of the sun on my skin brought a sense of renewal. The Sydney Adventist Hospital's location in Wahroonga, surrounded by greenery and bushland, made stepping outside feel like entering a peaceful sanctuary. I was profoundly grateful for that moment of freedom and connection with nature.

My friend Ronaldo, who is a hospital wardsman and someone I've known for a long time as a friend, came to visit me a few times during his shifts. It was nice to see a familiar friendly face in the staff. As a wardsman, Ronaldo takes care of all sorts of practical jobs on the ward, from moving patients and equipment to helping keep things running smoothly behind the scenes. His role is vital, often unnoticed but deeply appreciated by those who benefit from his steady presence. Ronaldo made a point of visiting me a couple of times during his night shifts, popping in quietly to say hello and check how I was holding up.

On one of his rounds, Ronaldo was joined by Chris, a nurse who quickly became one of my favourites. Chris is a gentle soul, always ready with a soft word and a reassuring smile. He'd looked after me in the ICU, and his visits to my room felt like little lifelines during the toughest nights. Chris had a knack for knowing when I needed comfort; one evening, noticing my anxiety before a new procedure, he took a moment to sit by my bed and talk me through what to expect, offering practical advice and calming my nerves. He told me he remembered me from my time in intensive care, and seeing how far I'd come filled him with genuine happiness.

Both Ronaldo and Chris went above and beyond their roles – Ronaldo with his quiet support and Chris with his attentive kindness. Their visits weren't just routine check-ins; they were moments that helped restore my spirit and made me feel less alone in an unfamiliar world. I'm deeply grateful for the comfort they brought during some of my most vulnerable days. Their presence reminded me that healing isn't just about medicine and procedures – it's also about the people who show up, with warmth and care, when you need it most.

One day, while my parents were visiting, our friend Eisha came by. Our families have been closely linked for years, and though Eisha is ten years younger and was closer to my sister, she has always treated me as her big sister. Her concern was palpable; she spent time massaging my legs to ease the discomfort, and caught up with my parents outside my room, exchanging news and laughter. In a heartfelt moment, I heard her compliment my parents on their health and remark to my dad that he was looking much healthier than her own father, Uncle Anuruddha, who had undergone some heart surgery not long ago. Her visit not only brought comfort but also strengthened the sense of family and history that has always supported me during challenging times.

Each visitor, whether family or friend, contributed to the fabric of my recovery. Their gestures – large and small – wove together a tapestry of care, compassion, and resilience, making the sterile hospital environment feel a little brighter each day.

The Hospital Room

When I was admitted to the Sydney Adventist Hospital, I requested a single room but had to share with another patient because the hospital was full.

My first roommate was an elderly Australian lady who had Parkinson's disease. One night, while I was asking for water, she tried to help by offering me some, not realising that I was not yet allowed to have thin fluids. The nurses became concerned. The elderly lady was only trying to be kind, but her well-intentioned gesture could have put me at risk. Eventually, she was moved out of Sydney to be closer to her family. I remember feeling a mix of gratitude for her kindness and anxiety about my own vulnerability in those early days, relying so much on the awareness of those around me.

After my first roommate left, I was placed with a 95-year-old lady of Hong Kong origin who had suffered a stroke. Her children were incredibly devoted, taking turns to sleep over and care for her. Witnessing their care made me reflect on the importance of family support during difficult times – it was both touching and reassuring to see such love in action. Their gentle attention to their mother, from adjusting her blankets to softly speaking to her in Cantonese, left a lasting impression on me. It made me think of my own parents and how their presence gave me strength throughout my recovery.

Later during my stay, I shared a room with another patient who was suffering greatly and often cried out in pain. Rest became almost impossible, and I found myself growing increasingly exhausted and overwhelmed. Eisha visited again that day and asked me why that patient was shouting so much. I told her I didn't know but I heard she had an infection or something so she must be in pain. Sensing how much this was affecting my recovery, Dr Roshni requested that I get moved to a single room so I could rest.

Each of these experiences – whether receiving a small gesture of help, witnessing unwavering family devotion, or being offered compassion by the hospital staff – shaped my journey and reminded me of the many forms care and kindness can take during times of hardship.

Overall, my stay at the Sydney Adventist Hospital was a positive experience. The staff did everything possible to make me comfortable, despite my condition.

Support from Family

My parents stayed in Sydney for three extra weeks to support me during my recovery. When the day arrived for them to leave, a wave of sadness washed over me. I knew I had to say goodbye and couldn't keep them with me any longer. That morning, I lingered on every word and every gesture, trying to hold onto the comfort and reassurance they brought. The thought of being without them made my recovery feel lonelier and more daunting.

Thankfully, my uncle Chandra had travelled from Germany the previous night to help with my recovery. Ravin had kindly helped with his airport pickup, which was a relief – I didn't want my elderly father driving all that way at night. My parents and Uncle Chandra overlapped by a day, giving us the chance to all be together, if only briefly. Knowing my uncle was in Sydney brought me immense relief. With his forty-five years as a nurse in Germany, I would be in good hands.

The morning Uncle Chandra arrived at the hospital, he was cheerful as always and with my parents. Nurse Helene, originally from Denmark, had just finished washing me – a challenging task that required two nurses due to my need for a mobility machine. Despite this, Helene was consistently cheerful and kind.

My uncle and parents greeted me warmly, and I managed to exchange a few words with them. Speaking was still a struggle – my voice sounded childlike, and each word required effort – but I was determined to connect with them despite my limitations.

I introduced my uncle to the hospital staff, and they welcomed him as a fellow healthcare professional. His warmth and experience quickly won their respect, and I felt proud to have him by my side.

My parents also became familiar faces to the staff. On the day they left for Perth, doctors Kim and Roshni, the physiotherapist, and several nurses gathered to say farewell. Their kindness and the sense of community made the moment bittersweet. As I watched my parents say goodbye to the hospital staff, I felt a deep gratitude for the support and compassion that had surrounded me – both from my family and the caregivers. The memory of their farewells lingers with me, a reminder of the strength that comes from being cared for and loved during life's most challenging moments.

After my uncle arrived, he visited me at the hospital every day. I introduced him to the staff and to my friends who came by. My friends Gerald and Dominic visited one day and brought me a book of Buddhist quotes as a gift. They were quite fond of my uncle and enjoyed their conversation with him.

Three weeks after the surgery, a few days after my uncle arrived, I was going to a rehabilitation hospital in Turramurra named Lady Davidson. By then I just started to walk using a frame.

After saying goodbye to the staff at the Sydney Adventist Hospital, I was placed in a patient transport vehicle destined for Lady Davidson. Until that moment, I'd always imagined patient transport vehicles were just ambulances. This one looked like an ambulance on the inside – complete with a little bed for me – but there was no blaring siren or urgent lights. The quiet, subdued atmosphere heightened my sense of transition: I was leaving one chapter behind and heading into the unknown.

Lying beside me was an elderly Lebanese lady, also being transported – her destination a nursing home along the same road as my rehabilitation hospital. She spoke softly, her voice tinged with both sadness and resignation. 'I was at the San for a few days because of some medical issue,' she shared, 'but now I'm heading back to the nursing home where I live.' As she talked about her situation, she confided that she wasn't happy to be there. 'After my husband passed away, my children put me in the nursing home because I needed medical attention,' she explained. Her gentle manner and openness made me reflect on how much one's circumstances can change after a loss.

The ride itself felt surreal and uncomfortable. The unfamiliar environment made me anxious, and I found myself wishing for the comfort of familiar faces. I gazed at the ceiling of the vehicle, trying to distract myself from the strange sensation of being in transit. My thoughts drifted between the kindness of hospital staff I'd just left behind and the uncertainty that awaited me.

Relief washed over me as we finally reached Turramurra. Once we arrived, the Lebanese lady was dropped off at the nursing home, while I continued to Lady Davidson, feeling both grateful that the journey was over and apprehensive about what lay ahead.

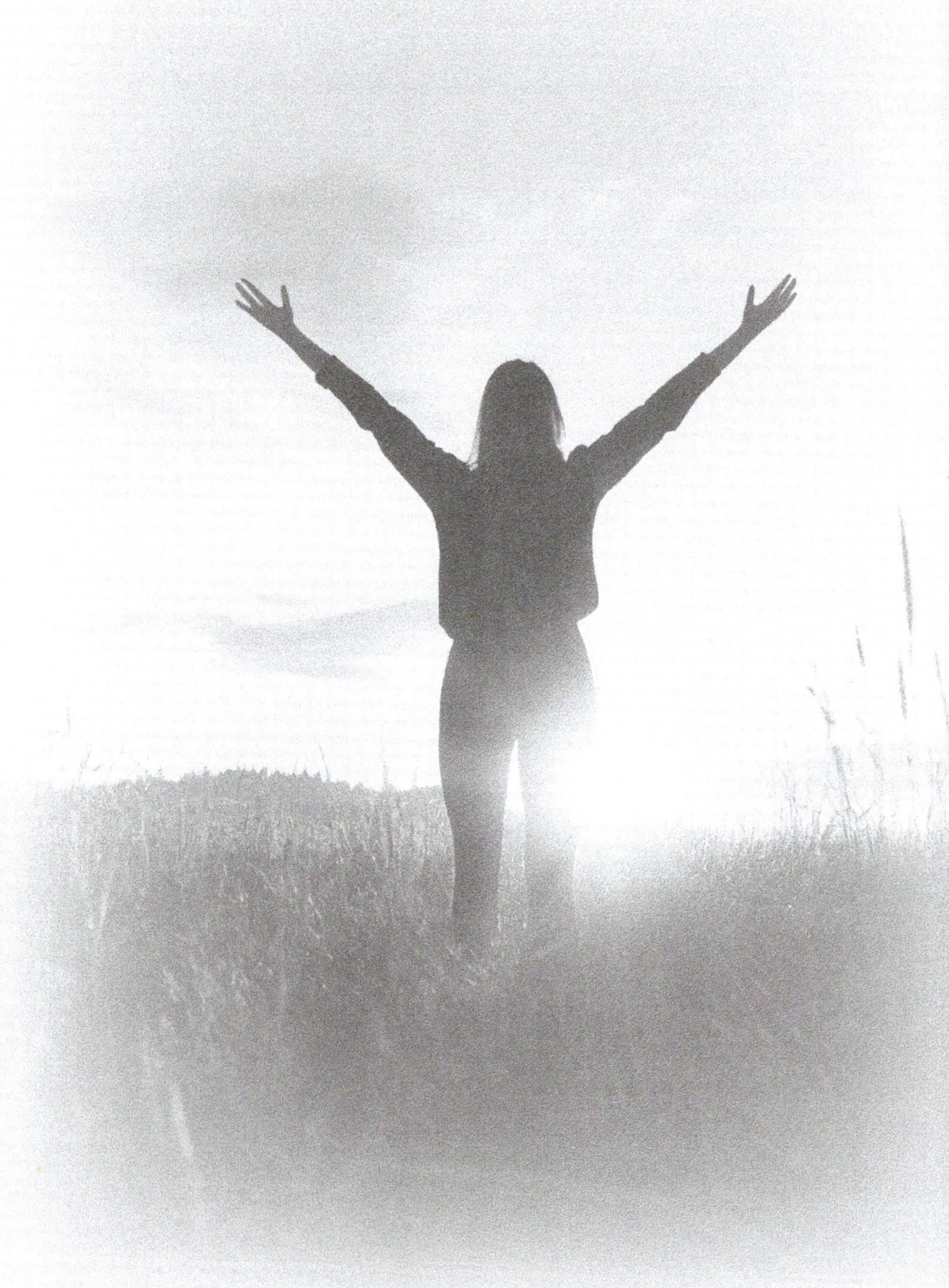

Chapter

5

Rehabilitation at Lady Davidson

Arrival and First Impressions

I was admitted to Lady Davidson Private Hospital in Turramurra at 2.00 pm on 7 November 2023, just a day shy of my sister's birthday – a detail that anchored the experience in memory. The timing of my arrival coincided with a staff shift change, so my introduction was met by a flurry of activity: a nurse and several student nurses welcomed me, their faces a mix of curiosity and concern. Some later admitted they initially thought I had cerebral palsy because I struggled to move, handle simple tasks, or speak clearly. That initial misunderstanding stung, but it also highlighted the vulnerability I felt – my identity overshadowed by visible limitations.

Lady Davidson, a private hospital dedicated to rehabilitation, immediately struck me as outdated and less than spotless. The facility's age was visible everywhere, and the halls seemed to echo with the shuffle of overworked staff. Most carers were students on placement – nurses, physiotherapists, and occupational therapists, all operating under minimal supervision. Their efforts were genuine and caring, but I sensed an undercurrent of exhaustion – a system under strain.

Despite these challenges, the team did their best to support my rehabilitation, greeting me each day with encouraging smiles that sometimes masked their fatigue.

Daily Life and Rehabilitation

Settling into my new routine, I quickly realised that my recovery would be slow and, at times, frustrating. The physiotherapist assigned to me was a final-year university student – confident and well-meaning yet bound by caution. 'I'm not allowed to let you walk or move much yet – we just can't risk a fall,' she explained, her tone gentle but firm. I understood her concern, but the restrictions left me feeling powerless. I spent hours staring at the ceiling, longing for movement beyond the confines of my room. Even a trip to the toilet required being ferried by staff on a small ride-on machine named Sara Steady, always dependent on someone else to propel me forward. My thoughts were often plagued by doubt: How will I ever walk again if I'm not allowed to try?

The highlight of each day was the hand therapy class run by the occupational therapists. These sessions became my sanctuary – a place to reclaim some agency. We worked through exercises designed to restore function to hands weakened by brain surgery. My left hand was particularly stubborn, plagued by pins and needles, as well as a persistent weakness that made even holding a pen a challenge – an especially cruel twist for someone left-handed. The group dynamic helped. Meeting others facing similar battles – some recovering from surgery, others from stroke – reminded me I wasn't alone. I struck up friendships with several of the older ladies, sharing stories as we fumbled our way through exercises together.

Still, as the days slipped by, I was getting depressed. There was not much progress when it came to walking, and the monotony of restricted movement weighed heavily on me. While my speech improved thanks to a dedicated speech pathologist – her encouragement and patience were a rare bright spot – my legs felt useless, and I worried that I would never reclaim my independence.

Moments with visitors became lifelines. My uncle and Brian came every afternoon around 5.30 pm, bringing not just home-cooked meals (courtesy of my uncle) but also an energy that chased away the institutional gloom. Brian, despite his demanding job, made the effort to sit by my bedside, share news from the outside world, and offer words of encouragement: 'Hang in there, you're tougher than you think.' Weekends brought other friends, each leaving their own mark on my journey. The laughter, the quiet chats, the simple companionship – they nourished a hope I'd begun to lose.

Life on the ward meant getting to know other patients and witnessing their struggles and triumphs. There was a man in his forties, always with a sombre air, who would brighten only when his young son visited on Sundays. He confided quietly, 'I just want to be home with my boy, but the landlord's dragging their heels on the house modifications.' Watching him play with his son, I felt a pang – wishing, for both our sakes, that recovery didn't have so many bureaucratic hurdles.

Another patient, a man in his fifties, took daily walks with crutches – each step a small victory. I watched him disappear down the hall with his wife by his side when the day came for his discharge. There was also an elderly Chinese lady who was recovering remarkably well from both cardiac surgery and a stroke. She walked with a frame, joined hand therapy, and taught me a few exercises. 'You must do this,' she insisted, gently guiding my fingers, 'it helped me.' When her daughter came to take her home to Ryde, she left with a smile and a wave, a gentle reminder that healing is possible.

But the departures, though hopeful for others, often deepened my own despair. One afternoon, I caught sight of someone walking outside my window and unexpectedly bursting into tears. The nurse who found me – her accent hinting at Nepal – sat by my side and quietly reassured me:

'Don't lose hope. It takes time, but it will get better.' Her words lingered long after, a thread of comfort I clung to in darker moments.

Discharge Process

After about a week, with progress still slow, I began to feel truly depressed. When I asked the doctor in charge and the chief nurse about going home, they cautioned, 'It could take months before you're ready.' The thought was unbearable – six weeks in hospitals already, my beloved cat still at the cattery, and no end in sight. My uncle, ever practical and reassuring, agreed: 'If you think you're ready, let's make it happen.' My sister, a social worker in Perth, became my advocate from afar, calling the hospital to request a walking frame and psychological support. I was granted only a single hour-long session with a psychologist, but it was something.

Determined, I asked my sister and Brian to help me find out if I could discharge myself. When they confirmed it was possible – even against medical advice – I informed the staff of my plan to leave by December 2023. Before I could go, the occupational therapists visited my home to assess its safety. With my uncle – a nurse with 45 years' experience in Germany – preparing to stay and care for me, they approved my discharge. They recommended a wheelchair and a portable toilet chair, estimating a cost of about $1000 even with a NDIS claim. My uncle was sceptical about their necessity, but I purchased them anyway – better safe than sorry.

Reflections: Resilience Forged in Uncertainty

Looking back, my time at Lady Davidson tested me in ways I never expected. The restrictions, the slow progress, and the ever-present frustration often threatened to drown out hope. Yet, through the kindness of visitors, the camaraderie among patients, and the unwavering support of family and friends, I found the resilience to keep going. Moments of sadness were tempered by laughter in hand therapy, and despair gave way to determination as I watched others take their hard-won first steps toward independence. The journey was not linear, nor was it easy, but each encounter – every conversation, every small gesture – reminded me that recovery is as much about community and compassion as it is about medicine. I left Lady Davidson changed: not just physically, but with a deeper appreciation for perseverance, empathy, and the quiet strength that emerges when hope feels most fragile.

Chapter

6

Homecoming

My uncle and Ravin picked me up from the rehabilitation hospital on 1 December 2023 and finally I came home. It was such a relief to be home after two months in hospitals. I still couldn't walk, as I was not encouraged to practise at the rehabilitation hospital. However, from the second day after coming home, with my uncle's help, I started to walk.

First my uncle held my hand as I walked around the block. I was scared to walk, thinking I would fall; that was what they told me at the rehabilitation hospital. But my uncle encouraged me. He always thought I could walk, so I got more confident. We returned the wheelchair and other equipment we purchased at the hospital. Just as my uncle thought, I did not need them. We went to mobility shops and hired various walking frames – however, as my left hand was still weak, it was difficult to push the frames, and we had to return them.

One day, we thought we would see if a stick would help me to walk. We found an old mop and went for a walk carrying that. My neighbours saw this and wondered what was going on. Only this couple I knew from upstairs, Maureen and Marten, knew I underwent major surgery. The others didn't know. So, I told them and introduced my uncle to them. I also told the caretaker lady of the apartment block about what happened.

After two days at home, my cousin Lalanthi from Melbourne came to visit us for a week. That was nice, as she was one of the other nieces of my uncle. During her stay, she took over the cooking and some of the housework. I could not yet do anything, and my uncle had to do everything, so I was relieved my cousin came to help. She is an excellent cook, so we did not mind her taking over meals.

The cattery dropped Archie home the day my cousin came and I was thrilled to see him after so long. That was the longest separation of Archie and me, but he was well looked after, and he settled well into his home again. I introduced him to my uncle and cousin, who both love animals. They were playing with Archie and were happy to meet him.

My cousin stayed for a week and during that time we laughed so much, and she cooked various recipes for us. One day my uncle and cousin went shopping and bought ingredients to make Sri Lankan cutlis, wade and curries. We all enjoyed that. I still couldn't taste well as the nerves were damaged, but even I enjoyed the food.

After a week, with Ravin's help, we dropped my cousin at the airport. She said a sad farewell to both of us, especially to our uncle, as she didn't know when she would see him again. She would see me again soon but once our uncle returned to Germany, it would be difficult to see him. It was nice to have my cousin over.

Every day my uncle and I went for a walk. Eventually I walked with a walking stick and even managed to climb stairs. With my uncle's patience and guidance, my walking was improving. One day Eisha came and the three of us went to Wahroonga for a walk. That was pleasant as Eisha also helped me with the walk. She is a fitness instructor and has experience helping older people who had strokes; she knew how to help me with any balance issues. We were chatting and laughing while we walked. It was a huge, pleasant change from the rehabilitation hospital. I was so glad to be home with loved ones.

During our daily walks along the sun-dappled footpath, my uncle gently guided me as I shuffled forward, each step an anxious effort. The air often carried the soft scent of eucalyptus from the nearby park, and the distant hum of traffic mingled with birdsong overhead. An old Chinese gentleman – stooped and silver-haired, his eyes warm and gentle – lived in the next street. He used to sweep leaves off his driveway daily. At first, he watched quietly from his driveway as I struggled with each uncertain step, his hands folded patiently behind his back. His encouraging smile, framed by deeply etched lines, offered silent support in the early days when my confidence wavered and my legs trembled.

As the weeks passed and my stride grew steadier, I noticed his greetings became brighter – his gentle eyes would crinkle with delight, and his slow, deliberate wave grew more enthusiastic. Some mornings, the breeze rustled leaves from overhanging branches, and he would gesture towards them as if sharing their beauty with me. Though he spoke little English, his presence was a daily encouragement, and I felt a comforting sense of companionship in his silent cheer. Each time our paths crossed, I was reminded of how far I'd come, and the warmth of this quiet, wordless friendship made the journey feel a little easier.

Each day, I could feel my walking getting stronger. Mornings began with dedicated routines – my uncle guiding me through exercises for my hands and legs, patiently encouraging each movement. For my eyes, he devised vision drills to address my double vision, gently reminding me to focus and persevere. He urged me to sing and read aloud, saying it would help regain my voice. Holding a pen, practising my writing, and even attempting to draw became small daily victories, each action helping to restore the dexterity in my left hand.

After the morning therapy routine, the kitchen would fill with the aroma of sizzling prawns and fresh avocados. My uncle lovingly prepared meals, explaining how ingredients like fish, walnuts, and leafy greens were especially good for my brain's recovery. Every morning, he would boil water and use it to massage my left leg and arm, the warmth easing stiffness and pain. His dedication was unwavering; he even brought special tools from Germany to help improve my hand grip, always thinking ahead and adapting the exercises as I progressed.

It couldn't have been easy for him to witness his niece enduring such hardship, but his determination to help only grew stronger. His love for both me and my mother (whom he is very close to) gave him the strength to support me through this journey. My parents and sister were eternally grateful for his care, and we spoke daily, drawing comfort from each other. The phone rarely stopped ringing as family members reached out with encouragement and support, reminding me I was never alone on this path.

Ravin and his friend Kristel visited often, sometimes bringing home-cooked Sri Lankan food. Kristel's housemate was a good cook so there was always something tasty to share.

Brian came over every day – sometimes bringing Sri Lankan short eats from the grocer nearby. The spicy aroma of fish cutlis mingled with the flaky texture of vegetable patties, filling the kitchen with warmth and stirring memories of home. The golden crust of the patties gleamed under the kitchen light, and the first bite always brought a burst of heat and spice that made my mouth water.

Since he speaks fluent German, Brian often waited until I was out of earshot before switching to German with my uncle – perhaps to give my uncle a chance to speak his native tongue without making me feel excluded. Although

I had studied German for two years, my skills were still lacking, so I often listened quietly as Brian and my uncle chatted in fluent German, sensing my uncle's comfort in using his native tongue.

My gym friends dropped by as well, and I loved introducing them to my uncle. He had a knack for making people feel welcome.

One afternoon, my Sri Lankan friends Rana, Viktoria, Siva, Clive and Dinali joined us for lunch in Five Dock, bringing a lively mix of stories and personalities to the table. Siva, always the storyteller about current affairs of Sri Lanka, recounted the latest news from Sri Lanka – his vivid descriptions of the political climate sparked a passionate discussion. Viktoria, who is a fitness instructor, was talking about healthy eating and shared a tip about using fresh turmeric for joint pain. The afternoon was filled with warmth, humour and the comfort of shared memories, making it a truly memorable gathering. Throughout lunch, my friends told me how rare it was to meet someone as selfless and kind as my uncle, and how lucky I was to have him by my side. Hearing their words, I realised how deeply his presence had changed my recovery – his sacrifice made me feel truly supported and cared for. Our relationship grew stronger with each passing day, and his unwavering commitment taught me what it means to show love through action.

One day, I had to see my GP Dr Fitzmaurice. When we arrived at the clinic, I introduced Uncle Chandra to Dr Fitzmaurice. The doctor's eyes immediately brightened, and a warm smile spread across his face as he saw me walking more steadily. He reached out and shook my uncle's hand, holding it firmly and expressing his gratitude by saying, 'Thank you for looking after Janani,' to Uncle Chandra for his care and support. Watching them interact, I felt a wave of relief wash over me – my uncle's face relaxed into a gentle smile, and his eyes lit up with quiet pride and kindness. Their handshake seemed to carry mutual respect and appreciation, and I was deeply moved to see those two important people in my life connect so sincerely. Later, as we left the clinic, Uncle Chandra confided that he liked my GP very much and thought I was in very good hands. His reassurance made me feel safe and grateful for the support surrounding me.

One day we hopped on a train to the city, to join some of my friends for our annual pre-Christmas dinner. The gentle hum of the carriage mingled with muffled announcements and the distant clang of city light rail, as we made our way towards the heart of Sydney. The city was alive with festive energy – streets lined with twinkling Christmas lights, and crowds of shoppers searching for Christmas gifts. At first it was difficult to find the restaurant. Mary, Deborah, Audrey and Carrie were already there, and when I arrived I told them it was not easy to find the place but finally someone on the street directed us to it. Despite my walking difficulties I was proud we still made it. They all said they got lost too, as the address was not very clear.

Our annual pre-Christmas catch-up is a tradition we've cherished for years – these wonderful ladies have been by my side for about twenty years, weaving themselves into the fabric of my life through celebrations, challenges, and everything in between. During tough times, these gatherings became my anchor, reminding me that I was never alone and that their support would always see me through. I can remember many dinners with them: each time we'd meet at a good restaurant, thanks to Mary who always found us a top spot at a fraction of the usual price using her Groupons. The air would be filled with the aroma of delicious food, and the sound of our laughter echoing in the lobby always signalled the start of a memorable night.

In previous years, after dinner, we'd walk through the city to see the Christmas tree at Martin Place and the decorations at the David Jones shop windows. Unlike previous years when we'd marvel at the sparkling Christmas lights of the tree and the pretty David Jones window display, this time we stayed indoors. My legs still weren't up for long walks, and the drizzle outside meant it was best to remain inside, enjoying each other's company.

First, we all met at the restaurant lobby and exchanged hugs, the warmth of their embrace making me feel instantly at home. I introduced Uncle Chandra to them, and they all really liked him. The atmosphere was alive with anticipation, friendship and the gentle hum of conversation as we settled in. Uncle Chandra then said he was going to explore the city and would get something to eat somewhere else while we all caught up. He went to Circular Quay, leaving us to share stories, laughter, and the comfort of tradition. We asked him to join us, but he said he wanted to see the city while we were here. The last time he was in Sydney was in 2013 and this visit was not a holiday. I thought it was a good idea to let him enjoy our beautiful city at his own pace, so I said we would meet in two hours in the hotel lobby and he left.

We took the lift to the restaurant. A table near the window waited for us. As we settled in, soft music drifted through the air, and the aroma of delicious food promised a good meal ahead.

The restaurant was in the Circular Quay area, somewhere near the Four Seasons Hotel, so the surrounding scenery of Sydney Harbour was beautiful. Through the glass, I saw the city skyline sparkling with thousands of twinkling lights. It created a breathtaking view against the dark night sky. The festive atmosphere was alive with gentle conversation and bursts of laughter. The sound of glasses clinking mingled with the hum of voices, wrapping me in a sense of belonging.

Sitting there, I breathed in the holiday spices. Warmth from my friends' embraces reminded me just how deeply these friendships have shaped my life.

As I glanced around the table, a rush of memories filled me – especially of last year's Christmas catch-up, when we sat up late, trading stories well into the night. Each moment spent with these wonderful friends adds another layer to the history we share, and I silently vowed to hold onto these memories for years to come. It struck me how each of us has our own way of preserving these moments – some through stories, others through small traditions.

For Carrie, it's her camera that keeps the past alive. She was, as always, snapping photos of every smile and every plate of food. We all teased her for never putting the camera down, but secretly I was glad. Carrie's photos have become a precious record, especially during my recovery, helping me remember the laughter and warmth that carried me through tough times. Her enthusiasm behind the lens reminded me that gratitude isn't just a feeling – it's something we keep in stories, photos, and the company of old friends.

On New Year's Eve, a few of us went to Hornsby RSL Club to have dinner and I ended up with food poisoning the next day. Uncle Chandra told me not to take any medication, but to let it all out, which I did. He gave me ginger tea which helped. I couldn't eat anything but after one day I was better. Only I got food poisoning, probably as my body was weak.

Finally, it was the new year, and I was improving a lot. Now I could do household tasks such as cooking and I got a cleaner to tidy the house weekly. I was walking a lot better, and my speech was almost normal. The only problems I still had were tiredness and balance issues.

By the third month after my surgery, I still couldn't work or drive. My employer continued to hold my job for me, giving me hope that I might eventually return, but I was uncertain about when that would be possible. During this time, I was paid sick leave, which provided some financial relief while I recovered. Meanwhile, my financial advisor, Werner, discovered that I could claim trauma insurance. He came to my place to help complete the forms, as I couldn't write, and organised the application for me. A few weeks later, I received a lump sum payment that would help support me for a while, giving me a sense of relief but also reminding me of my ongoing limitations.

At the same time, I felt anxious about my future and uncertain whether I would ever regain my independence. The idea of ending my career early at 54 filled me with disappointment – I had always planned to retire at 65, and it felt too soon to be considering such a major change as giving up a career I enjoyed. I realised how much my life had shifted in only a few months, and I grappled with questions about what lay ahead and whether I would ever get back to where I was before.

February arrived, and with it came the moment for Uncle Chandra to return to Germany. The thought of saying goodbye filled me with sadness, and I quietly asked if he could stay a bit longer. My parents also asked him if he could stay longer. However, Uncle Chandra explained that he had to go back. Although I was regaining my strength and could manage most tasks around the house, the prospect of being alone after months of support was daunting.

As I watched Uncle Chandra prepare to leave, the thought of facing my days alone felt overwhelming – until Mary and Kathleen stepped in with their generous offer to stay at my place a week each after my uncle left, easing my anxiety. I realised just how much I'd come to rely on the comfort of having someone nearby, especially after spending three months with my uncle and two months in hospital before that. The fear of solitude had crept in, making my recovery seem more challenging.

Mary's optimism has a way of lifting everyone's spirits, and her knack for finding solutions, big or small, always reassures me. Kathleen, my oldest friend, rearranged her family commitments without hesitation. She made sure her son Liam was with his father for the week and took leave from work so she could be by my side. Both women have long been pillars in my life, offering unwavering support and genuine care.

The knowledge that Mary and Kathleen would take turns staying with me for two weeks brought a deep sense of relief. Their presence promised not only practical help, but also the companionship I needed to navigate the transition from constant support to greater independence. In that moment, I felt grateful comforted by the kindness of friends who step in when it matters most.

Finally, it was the day before my uncle left. We both felt very sad to say farewell. That night my uncle gave me a big hug and told me I would be alright with time, and he had tears in his eyes. My uncle is an angel in disguise.

A few days earlier, Peter and Diow invited my uncle, Dominic, Gerald and Joan and me to their place to lunch to say a farewell to my uncle. We gave my uncle a few gifts to remember Australia. As my uncle loves Australian flora and fauna, the gifts consisted of books and some prints on those topics. My friends said a farewell to my uncle and thanked him for coming here to take care of me.

On the day my uncle left, Ravin and I sent him off after a sad goodbye. Brian came the day before and bid farewell to my uncle too. I felt very sad but was so thankful to Uncle Chandra for his help; I said to him if he ever needed anything, to let me know.

That afternoon, Mary came to stay with me for a week. One day, we travelled to Hornsby for my acupuncture and other appointments. Afterwards, we enjoyed a relaxed lunch at a bustling café – the clatter of dishes and quiet chatter in the background made the time together feel cosy. Another day, the house was filled with the mouth-watering aroma of ginger and garlic as Mary cooked a Chinese meal for us. Every day we set out for a walk, feeling the cool air on our faces and listening to the soft rustle of leaves underfoot.

One day, Mary drove us to Dee Why so that we could see the ocean, which I hadn't seen in a while. The salty breeze, the rhythmic crash of the waves, and the endless blue horizon left us both feeling refreshed and uplifted. Even Archie took a liking to Mary, rubbing his tail around Mary's legs to show that she now belongs to him. This made me appreciate her company even more.

A week after Mary left, Kathleen arrived. Our days were spent much like before – taking daily walks, sometimes heading to Hornsby, or simply staying home to chat. Kathleen's company was delightful, and Archie enjoyed having her around too.

Once Kathleen departed a week later, I found myself alone with Archie. It felt strange at first, but I soon adjusted. My health had improved significantly, allowing me to resume my daily walks. When it came time for my brain surgeon appointment, Brian accompanied me. Dr Kim gave me a comprehensive check-up and was pleased with my progress, especially that I could walk unaided. He even filmed a video of me to share with Dr Roshni. I mentioned Dr Roshni's kindness, and Dr Kim agreed warmly, calling her 'a good egg'.

Afterwards, my routine included daily walks, weekly acupuncture sessions, and remedial massages. Gradually, I became more active, though I still wasn't well enough to drive or undertake long walks. Instead, I used taxis, trains, or accepted lifts from friends. The kind Chinese gentleman from the next street noticed my improvement and, several months later, was so overjoyed he crossed the road to give me a hug. The world needs more people like him – someone who celebrates a stranger's progress.

Recent global developments have highlighted immigration as a significant topic in many countries, including Australia. I have reflected on my own status as an immigrant, as well as that of most of my friends, and even several medical professionals – such as my brain surgeon and the many nurses who have treated me. Additionally, even that friendly elderly Chinese gentleman is an immigrant. These experiences lead me to believe that the presence of immigrants greatly contributes to the quality of life in our society, so I couldn't understand the big deal.

During this period, after my doctors gave their approval, I took a flight to Perth to visit my family. Being surrounded by loved ones lifted my spirits, and seeing their relief at my progress was heartening. In Perth, I enjoyed daily walks –

thanks to the city's flat terrain, getting around was easier and less tiring. Behind my parents' house, a peaceful park waited each morning. The soft grass beneath my feet, the scent of eucalyptus in the air, and the cheerful calls of native birds made every stroll a gentle pleasure.

I reconnected with my oldest friends – Celine, Naeim, and Shahla – sharing stories and laughter as we caught up on each other's lives. I also spent time with many family friends. During my stay, I visited priests and nuns from the local Buddhist Society of Western Australia, and their daily prayers for my recovery warmed my heart. Each meeting felt comforting, surrounded by kindness, familiar faces, and gentle encouragement.

After spending a month in Perth focusing on recovery and reconnecting with loved ones, I returned home feeling renewed and thankful for everyone's support. My efforts to improve my fatigue and balance continued.

However, after several weeks, I noticed my right eye was worsening and beginning to droop, prompting a visit to an ophthalmologist. Knowing my surgical history, he suggested I get an MRI and see my brain surgeon again.

The scan showed that the tumour had resumed growing in a part of my brain that couldn't be reached during the previous surgery. Dismayed, I shared the news with my family and friends before arranging another appointment with Dr Kim. Brian came along for the consultation, and my friend Nilmini kindly drove me home afterwards.

Dr Kim confirmed the recurrence of the tumour and recommended radiation therapy to address the new growth and reduce the risk of further regrowth. He referred me to Dr Cecilia Gzell, a radiation oncologist, with whom I scheduled a timely consultation. Although I initially experienced apprehension, Dr Kim's thorough explanations and reassurance regarding the effectiveness of radiation therapy alleviated my concerns about future recurrence. Brian accompanied me to these appointments and provided significant support during this period.

Chapter

7

Radiation Therapy

During my first consultation, Dr Cecilia Gzell explained that I would need to undergo a month-long course of radiation therapy to prevent the tumour from regrowing. She mentioned that a custom-fitted mask would be made for my head and face to keep me still during each session. The total cost of radiation was $40,000, which Medicare covered – making me appreciate how my years of paying taxes were now benefiting me.

Dr Gzell explained the medical procedure and side effects very well. Both Brian and I were very impressed with her knowledge. I saw not only did she have medical degree, but she also had a doctorate in medicine. I thought of her as a 'walking brain'. Dr Gzell reassured me that the main side effects would likely be fatigue, dry skin, and dry hair, stressing the importance of hydration and rest throughout the treatment period. I was relieved when she assured me that I wouldn't lose my hair.

Once the mask was ready, I began radiation therapy at Sydney Adventist Hospital, attending sessions every weekday for a month.

Since I was unable to drive and lived alone, I relied heavily on friends for transportation. Each session lasted about half an hour, and because the appointments were on weekdays, I chose not to disturb Brian, who had a demanding senior manager role. Instead, several retired or non-working friends generously helped. I reached out to Council Community Support but was informed that their services are only available to individuals over the age of 60. Subsequently, I learned about additional council support options available for a nominal fee, including access to nursing services, carers, gardening assistance, and cleaning services for individuals who are unwell and living alone.

In the first two weeks, Nilmini, Frank, and Deborah drove me to Norwest Hospital, about half an hour from home. I appreciated their help, as the hospital was far for all of us; they waited nearby at a café during my procedures. Each session lasted ten minutes, but the entire process took thirty due to mask fitting.

The radiation technicians played music while I was undergoing radiation – I guess they did that to calm my nerves. That was nice of them. On the first day they were playing Eric Clapton's 'Tears in Heaven'. Later I told them that was a sad song to play to a patient undergoing radiation for a terminal illness, and they agreed. Then they asked me what sort of songs or musicians I like. I'm a 1980s kid, so I love anything from the 80s. For the remainder of my radiation sessions, they played happier songs by my favourite artists. On the second day, to my delight, they played George Michael, who is one of my all-time favourites.

I received the last two weeks of radiation at the Sydney Adventist Hospital, just ten minutes from home. In the third week, my friend Ariel, whom I met two years prior at gym classes, adjusted her schedule to be with me during treatment. Although we hadn't known each other long, her kindness meant a lot. When I met her visiting parents from China at Christmas, I complimented them on raising such a caring daughter. Their visit also reminded me of my own unfulfilled wish for children, making me feel a bit sad. Ariel stayed at my flat during the final two weeks of radiation.

During my last week, I relied on Ganesh and Narend – two taxi drivers I've known for around twenty years – to get me to my appointments. I truly appreciated their help, and it was clear they cared about my wellbeing.

The actual process of radiation wasn't painful, but having to remain perfectly still as the machine operated was uncomfortable. Most days, I coped well once back home, though I vomited twice; thankfully, Ariel was there to support me during that time. The treatment left my skin and hair extremely dry, and I experienced severe exhaustion for weeks. Dr Gzell reassured me that these symptoms were expected and that my energy would gradually return.

Radiation therapy began to shrink what remained of the tumour and slow its regrowth. Dr Gzell was encouraged by the results shown in MRI scans before and after treatment, advising I return for follow-up visits every six months. She explained that improvements might continue for as long as twenty years. Dr Gzell also assured me I will not have to undergo surgery again – I was relieved.

Chapter

8

Another Christmas

After several months, my fatigue lessened, my eyesight improved, and the drooping eyelid gradually opened enough for me to drive again. Though it had now been a year since surgery and three months since radiation, I was still unable to work.

My employer kept my position open for a year, and until February 2024 I received paid sick leave, exhausting all annual leave in the process. By October 2024 it became clear that I couldn't return to my previous job due to health issues, so we mutually agreed on my resignation. Around that time, I received a trauma insurance payment from my superannuation fund; unfortunately, I didn't qualify for income protection, as it only covers accident-related health problems. Receiving trauma insurance was a relief since I can't access my superannuation until I turn 60, four years from now. In response, I sold my property in Wahroonga, settled my loans, bought a smaller property nearby in Waitara, and replaced my car with a more affordable one – practical decisions that have genuinely helped me.

My droopy eyelid improved significantly as months passed by – so, with the approval from both my optometrist and ophthalmologist, I resumed driving one year after surgery, starting with lessons to rebuild my confidence. At first, it felt unfamiliar, but over time I was able to drive locally, further distances, and at night. Now I enjoy driving my new car, though I have yet to drive on motorways or long trips as I'm not fully comfortable. I hope to gain enough confidence for long-distance driving soon.

Christmas came around again, and this year I felt noticeably stronger than the last. After my annual pre-Christmas gathering with Mary, Carrie, Audrey and Deb, we ventured into the city to see the Christmas lights. The city sparkled with strings of golden and crimson lights draped across shopfronts and trees, casting a warm, festive glow over the streets. Standing there among the crowds, I felt a mix of nostalgia and hope – grateful for how far I'd come since my treatment, and quietly optimistic about the year ahead.

I travelled to Perth to spend Christmas with my family. It was comforting to be together again, sharing laughter and stories at our usual family Christmas gathering at my sister's place. This year, Ravin and another friend, Arjan – whom I met through Rana years ago – also came to Perth for a holiday, so we invited them to our Boxing Day lunch, a tradition where friends join our family celebration. Celine, her kids, and her mum, Aunty Betty, were also there. Aunty Betty, now in her 90s, sat quietly among us. I remember first meeting her decades ago when she was lively and energetic, often playing badminton. Now, although she's still in good health for her age, she appears frail, a gentle reminder of how time moves on for all of us.

Looking around at my parents, Aunty Betty, and the rest of my family, I realised how precious these gatherings are. It struck me that we're all growing older, and these moments together are not to be taken for granted. I promised myself to call my parents more often, to visit whenever I could, and to cherish these simple celebrations while we still have them. Life moves quickly, and I want to make the most of every chance to be with the people I love.

I celebrated New Year's Eve to bring in 2025 in Perth with my family and then came back to Sydney few days later.

After following Dr Gzell's advice, I had a checkup at six months post-radiation (February 2025) with Brian. She was pleased – the tumour had stopped growing. She advised another checkup in six months. In August 2025, I went alone and learned the tumour was now shrinking, so appointments moved to once a year. My walking and vision improved, and both my doctor and I are satisfied with my recovery. I'm grateful to Dr Gzell for her expertise and clear explanations.

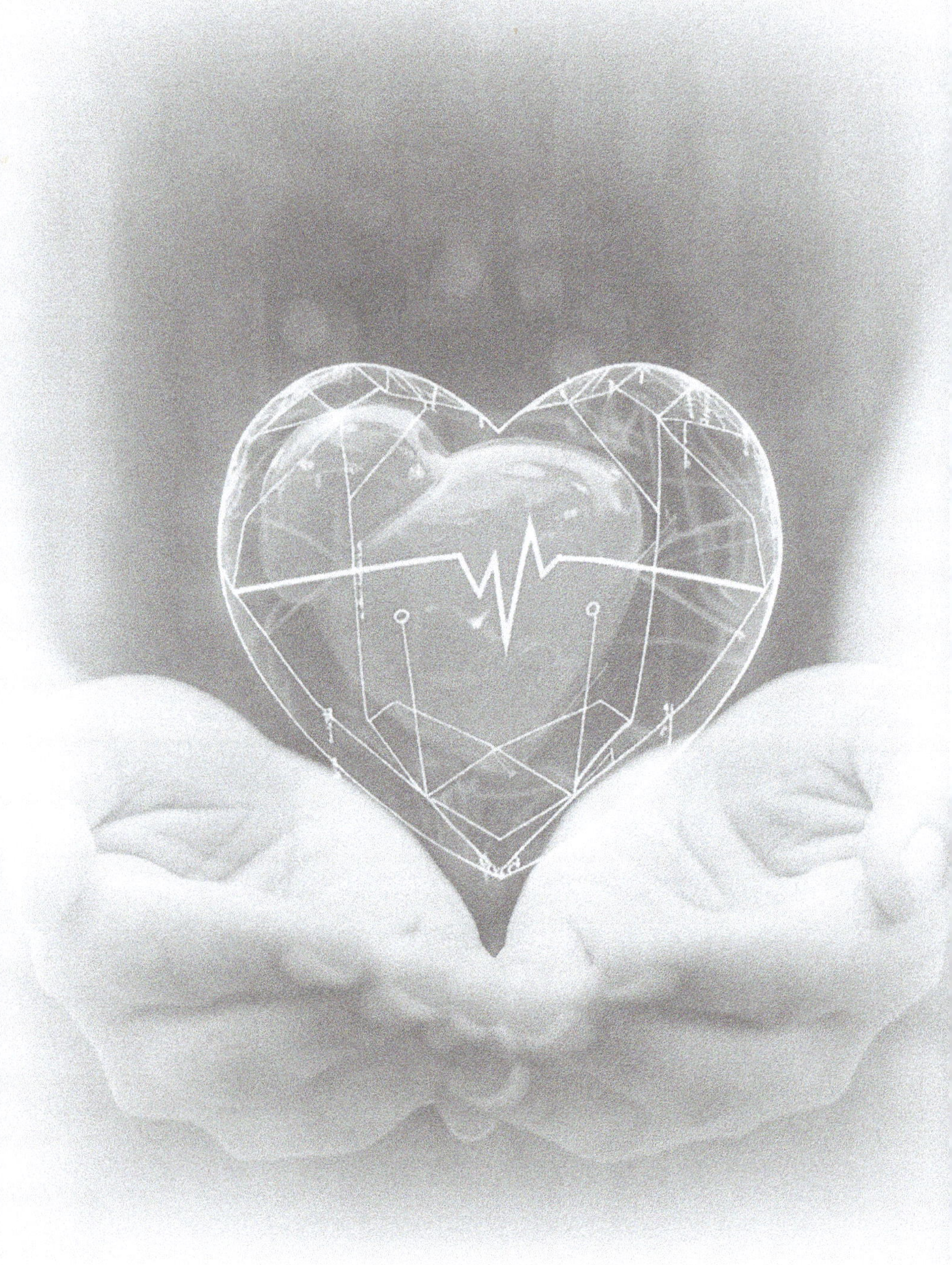

Chapter

9

Life after a Brain Tumour

Two and a half years later, I find myself making steady progress in my recovery. My ability to walk, talk, and see has noticeably improved, and my energy levels are improving. My sense of taste is returning, allowing me to appreciate food again. I can also drive small distances again.

Despite these positive changes, I am still not fully recovered. I would say I am a work in progress. I continue to experience balance issues and struggle with brain fog, which makes it difficult to concentrate. Bright lights from shopping centres, offices, or computer monitors still overwhelm me. I suffer from peripheral neuropathy in my left hand and foot, a lingering effect of nerve regeneration which can take a long time to heal. I am hopeful that these symptoms will gradually improve.

As I am recovering, with my doctor's permission, I started gym classes and walks. I spent Easter break in Perth with my family and travelled to China in July 2025 with Mary, Carrie, and one of Mary's friends. I hadn't gone on an overseas holiday since 2017, so I really enjoyed that trip. Travelling showed me I could walk for hours and was regaining strength. I visited the Great Wall and Tiananmen Square, using a walking stick when needed. I had to use a wheelchair at Tianamen Squre, as it was a hot day and we walked a lot in that heat. I am thankful I can go to the gym and travel – things I used to enjoy before the surgery.

I attempted to return to work by taking on some freelance projects for consultants I knew. However, I soon realised that working in an office environment or spending long hours at a computer was not manageable for me, as I needed to take frequent naps and struggled with fatigue. So, I decided to step away from work altogether, as it is not good for my health or fair to the employer when I take a long time to complete a task.

Even writing this book took more than a year because I cannot write or type properly due to nerve issues. I had to take long breaks. It was also a traumatic project, as I had to relive the trauma while writing it. However, writing this experience helped mentally.

It is fair to say that my whole life changed at the age of 53 after my brain tumour surgery. I have to end my career as a regulatory scientist in the pharmaceutical industry. All of my working life, after graduating from university as a chemist, I felt I was contributing to society by helping people with illnesses to heal. I found that immensely gratifying. Now I feel as if I am not contributing to the world at all. It's a strange feeling, after having studied and worked all my adult life. I miss my colleagues too.

If I were to naturally retire in my sixties then I would have been ready for that. This happened to me without warning, and it's a new reality I have to adjust to. It is a strange feeling. I get up in the morning thinking, 'What can I do today?' I cannot do much, as I get brain fog after a few hours of concentration, needing a nap. My body aches everywhere due to inflammation and I am slow in doing everything. I don't even eat like I used to. It is frustrating but it is out of my control. All I can do is to listen to what my doctors say, live healthy and try to be positive. Two years ago, I could not even sit up, now I can do most things I could do before. I moved to a smaller property I can manage easily, that is walking distance from the local train station and shops. Most of my friends live around me too, which helps.

I now devote more time to hobbies and prioritise my wellbeing. I attend the gym as often as possible, participating in activities like yoga, Pilates and Zumba. The combination of dance and music in Zumba provide an enjoyable way to boost brain coordination and lift my spirits. I started to attend more Zumba party classes and found that I can manage to participate better, and my physical strength is improving each day. In November 2025 I went to the Gold Coast to attend a large 'party' Zumba class organised to celebrate a visit by Beto Pérez, the inventor of Zumba. I really enjoyed that.

Regular walks further improve my balance. I increased meditation too, as I found it helped to calm my mind. I even attended a meditation retreat while in Perth in December 2025.

Socialising with friends is an important part of my routine, significantly benefiting my mental health. Other hobbies I enjoy are art and photography. I want to do an art course and maybe exhibit a few works in the local art school.

I find myself replacing work with gym classes, writing slowly (I really have to say 'slowly' is the key word these days), socialising with friends, reading a book or going for a walk. I go to the shops but have to be careful with finances, as I don't work anymore or receive superannuation yet. I am currently living off savings, which makes me very nervous, as I never planned for this and always had an income. I did receive some insurance money at the beginning to last me for a couple of years, but I will not receive my superannuation for another four years, which makes me very nervous.

After a long recovery, life is returning to a new normal for me. I still face challenges. It is frustrting but I accepted that things have changed. Despite these difficulties, I am grateful to be alive and able to do most things as I did before. Many others in my meningioma support group share similar experiences – outwardly we may seem fine, but adapting to these changes isn't easy. Still, life goes on, and it could have been much worse. The tumour could have been in an inoperable section of the brain, or it could have been a malignant brain tumour that would have killed me instantly. I consider myself as lucky to be able to write this as a survivor; I will never take that for granted.

Reflection

Reflecting on my experiences over the past two years, I feel proud for persevering without letting myself fall into despair. After being diagnosed with the brain tumour, I saw two possible paths: sinking into depression and hopelessness, or finding the strength to keep going with hope. Initially, I believed this kind of situation would never happen to me. However, when it eventually did, my first reaction was fear. After that passed, I chose to accept reality and handle it as best as I could – by staying calm and avoiding panic.

As someone born and raised Buddhist, I have always taken life one day at a time, believing that hardships touch everyone – wealth cannot purchase good health. Facing a serious illness and coming close to death reinforced my understanding that life is fleeting and filled with suffering. Whether moments are good or bad, nothing lasts forever.

This journey has intensified my spirituality; I meditate more, attend meditation sessions regularly, and deepen my study of Buddhist teachings. Regardless of your faith or beliefs, grounding yourself spiritually during tough times can make a profound difference. During my darkest hours, I found compassion even for the tumour itself through meditation. When undergoing radiation treatment, I would ask the tumour not to return, wishing it no harm. Ajahn Brahmavamso, a Buddhist priest in Perth whom I admire, has taught that cultivating positive thoughts and compassion – even towards illness – can aid healing. As a chemist, I see how compassion during meditation generates beneficial chemicals that promote wellbeing. Ajahn Brahmavamso, formerly a theoretical physicist before becoming a monk, shares my scientific perspective and is an inspiring teacher whom I am grateful to know.

Another vital lesson I've learned is the value of true friends, family, and community, especially in difficult times. These connections, though always important, became even clearer to me during illness. Life is a precious gift, and we should never give up, even when it's tempting to do so. Drawing inspiration from resilient people like my friend Mary strengthens my own resolve. Spirituality is essential, and kindness often brings support when you least expect it.

I hope my story inspires anyone facing a crisis. I wrote this book for fellow meningioma brain tumour sufferers, sharing my journey to help them prepare for their own challenges. I have included below some information I found useful during this ordeal.

My wish for every reader is to be blessed with good health, loving relationships, and the support they need. Thank you for taking the time to read my story. Even if this helps one of you, I will be happy.

Useful Information

Meningioma Australia

A Facebook support group that helps by sharing information with fellow meningioma suffers/survivors.

Ajahn Brahmavamso

His talks and meditation on YouTube helps to calm the mind to keep things in perspective from a spiritual point of view.

Smiling Mind and Headspace

Meditation apps that help to find calming guided meditation.

Royal Australasian College of Surgeons

Help to find information on brain surgeons and other specialists (https://www.surgeons.org/).

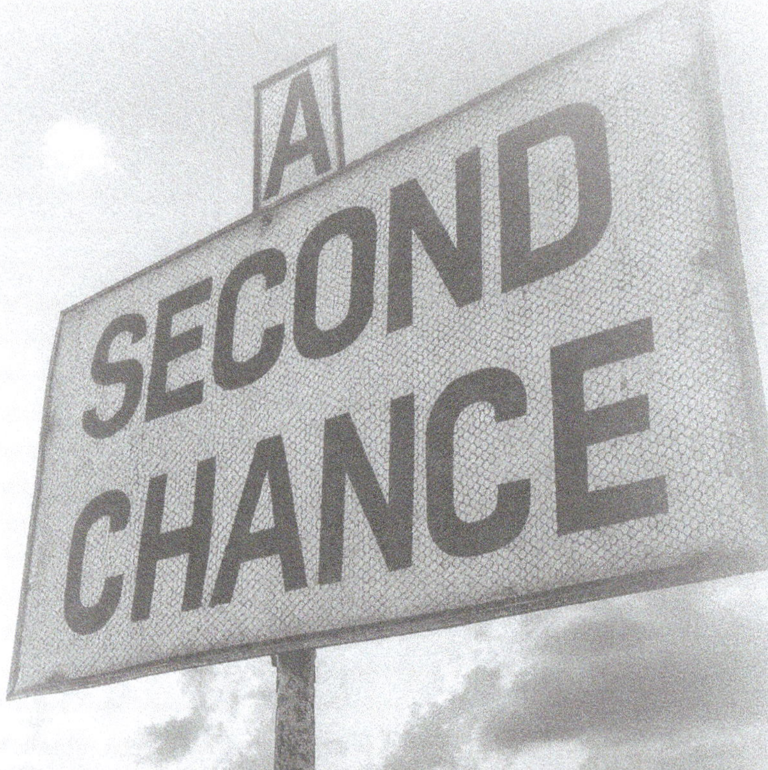

A
SECOND
CHANCE

About the Author

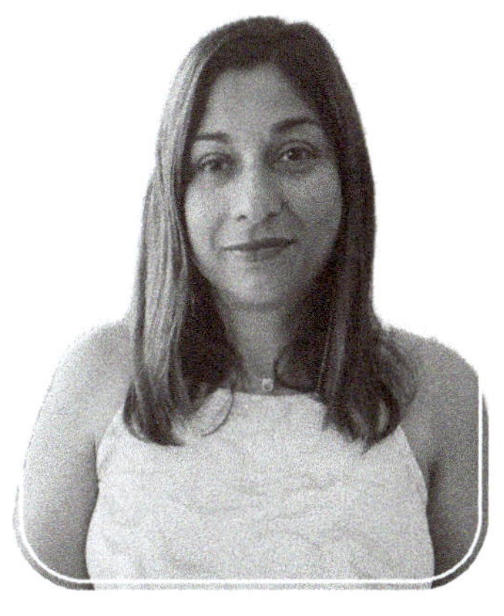

Janani Amarasuriya was born in 1969 in Sri Lanka. In 1982, she migrated to Australia with her parents and younger sister, beginning a new chapter of her life. Janani is a qualified chemist, having dedicated 30 years to working in the pharmaceutical industry. Her role as a regulatory scientist enabled her to contribute meaningfully to the field before she had to stop working due to illness. Janani now enjoys writing books and painting as hobbies. She leads a peaceful life in Sydney, Australia, sharing her home with her beloved cat, Archie.

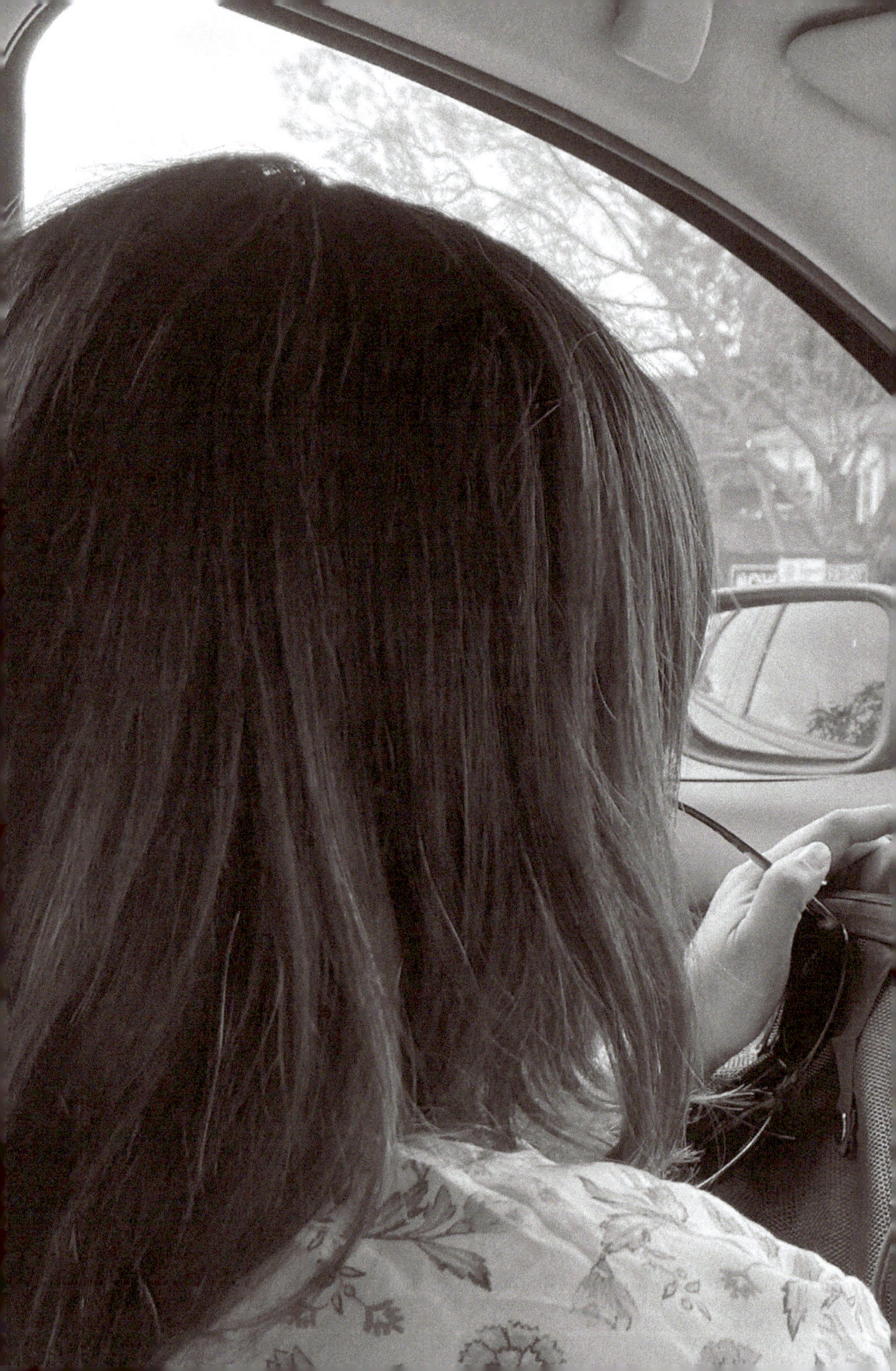

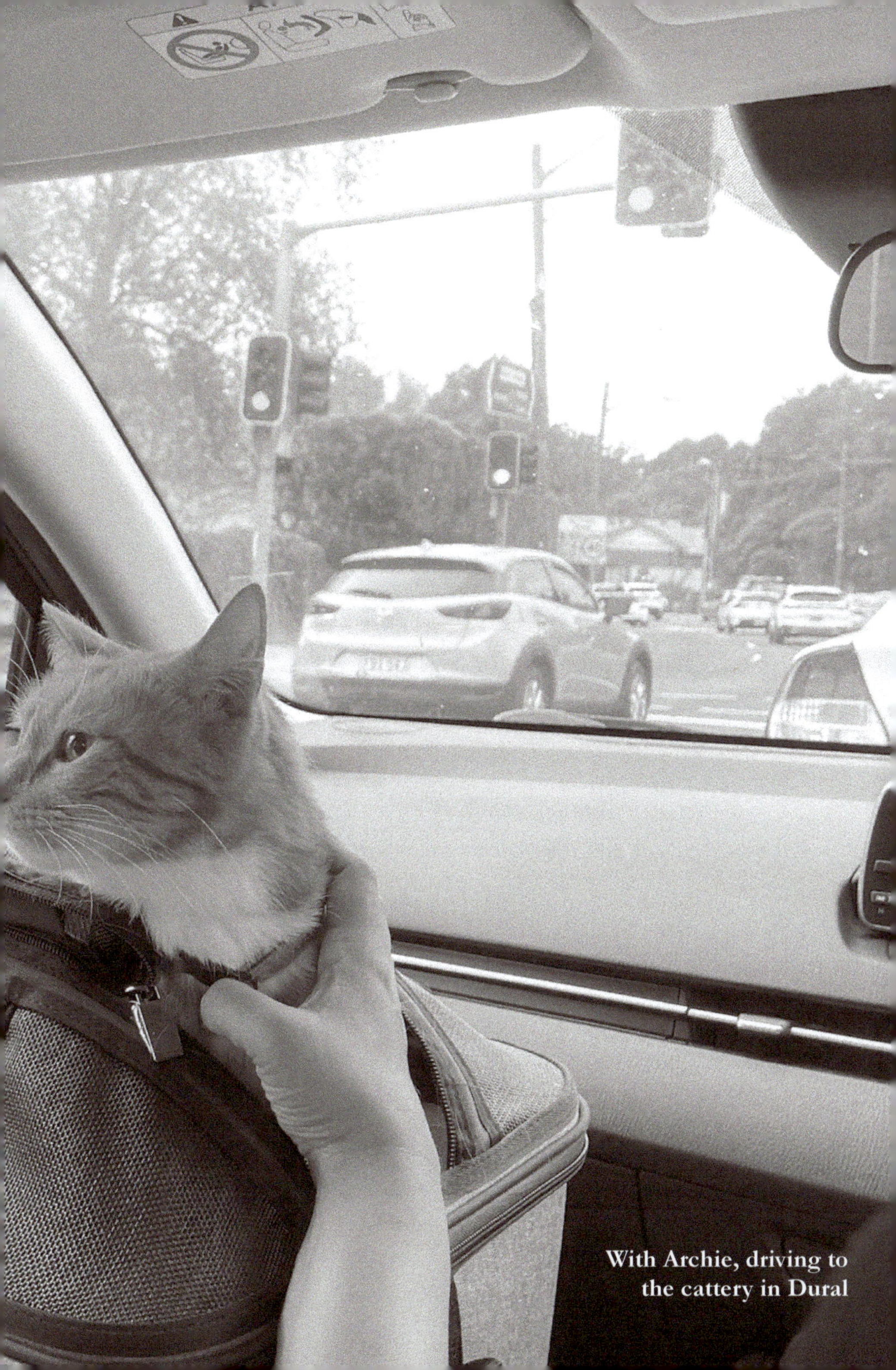

With Archie, driving to
the cattery in Dural

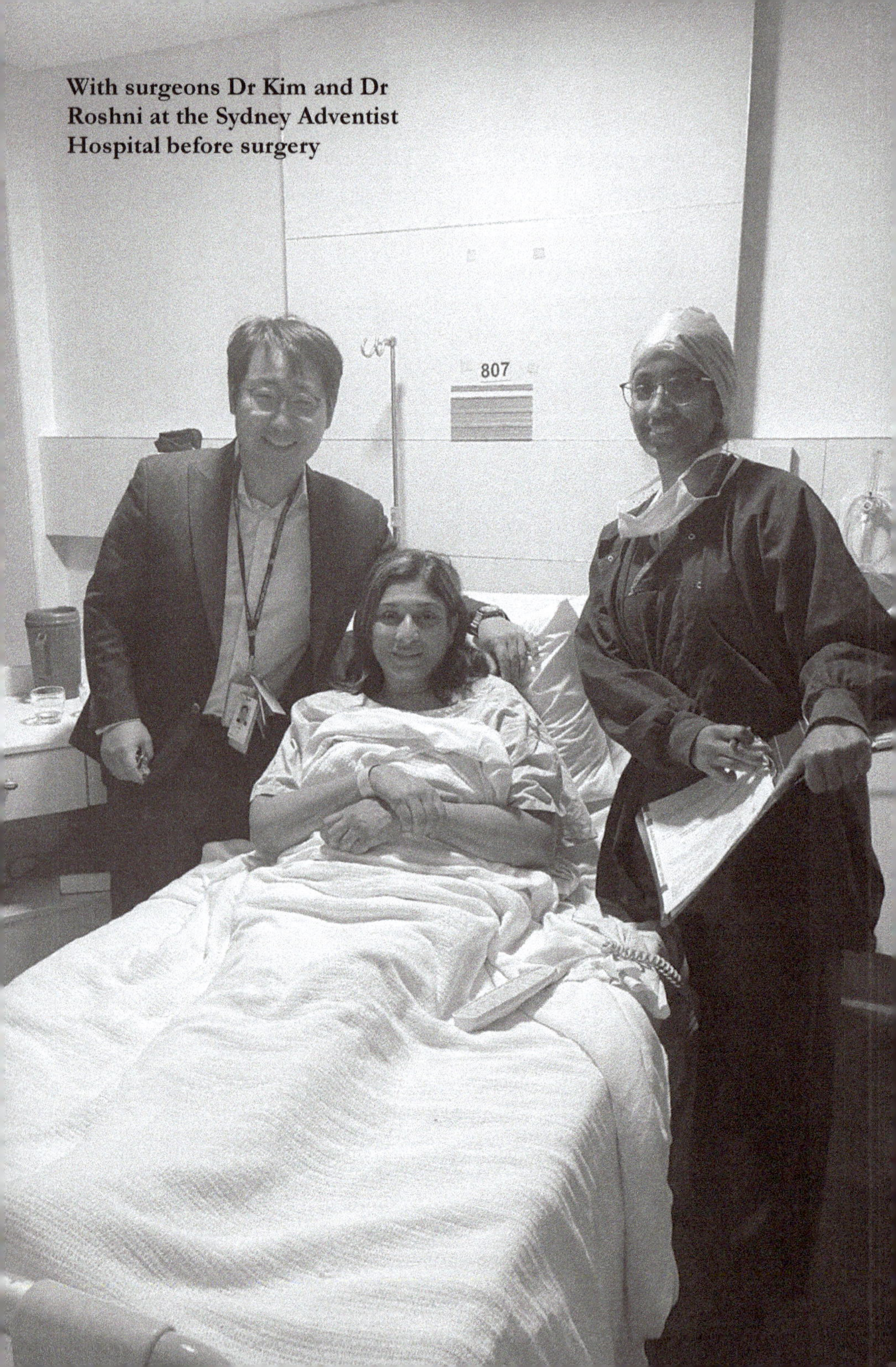

With surgeons Dr Kim and Dr Roshni at the Sydney Adventist Hospital before surgery

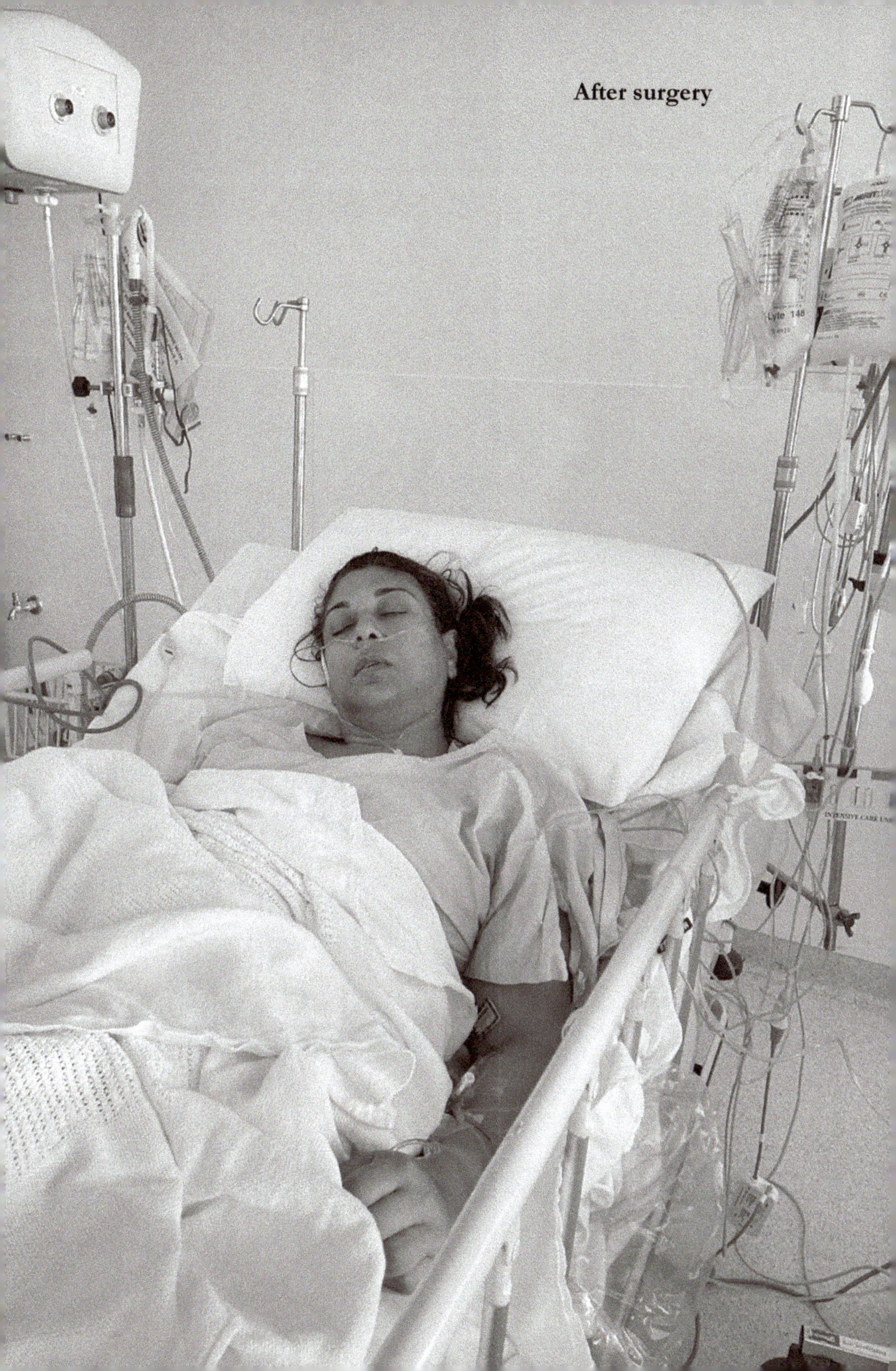
After surgery

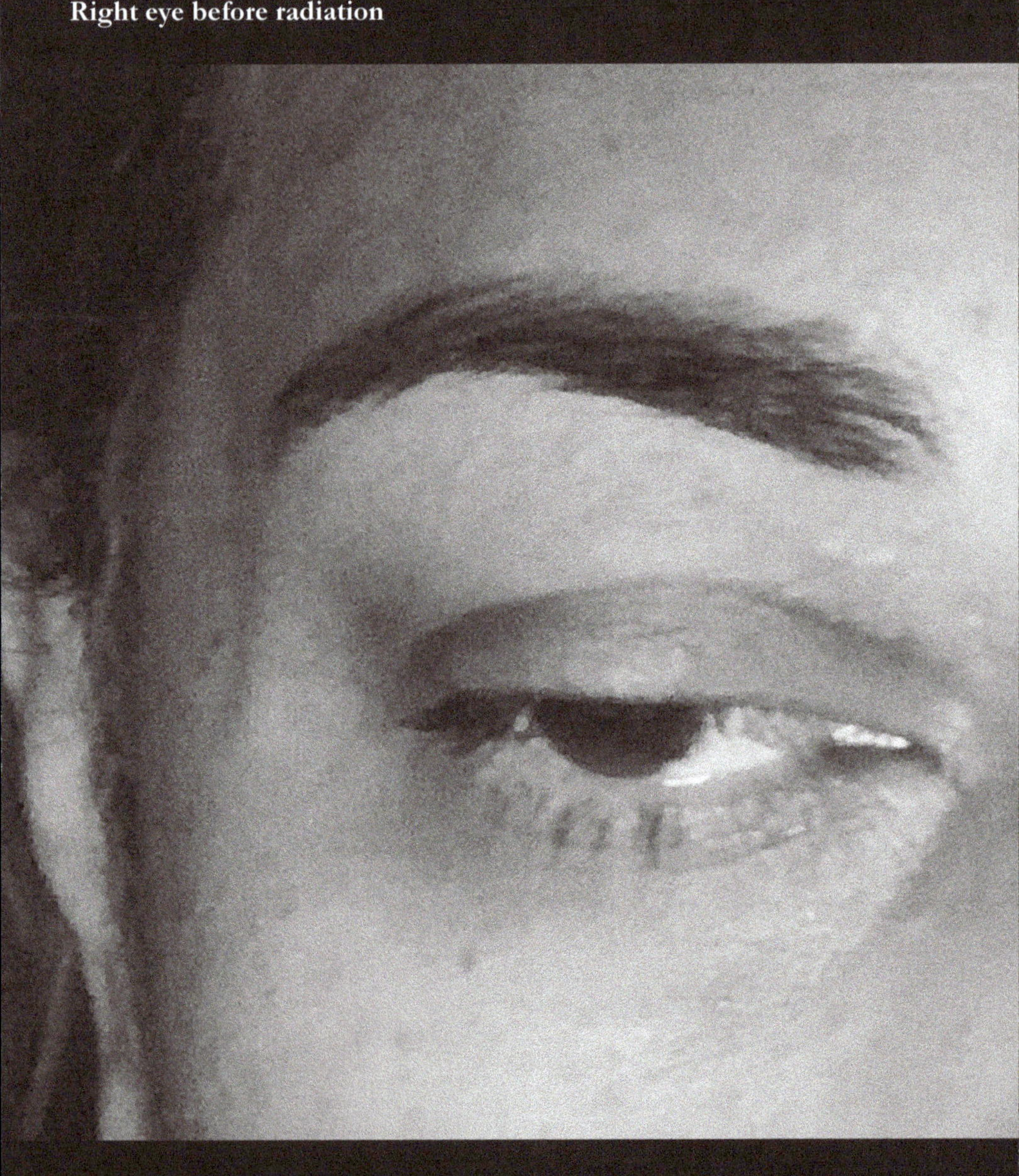

Right eye before radiation

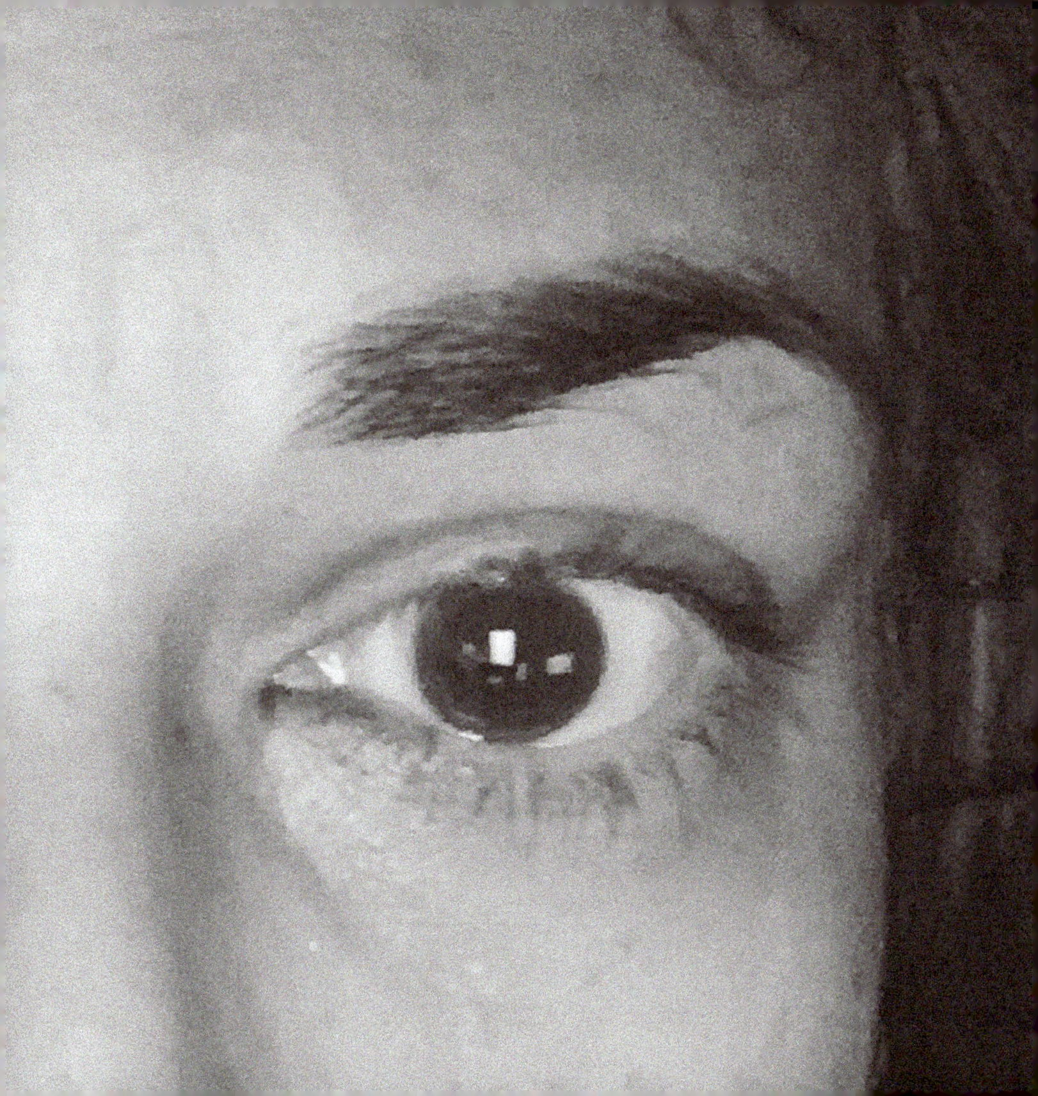

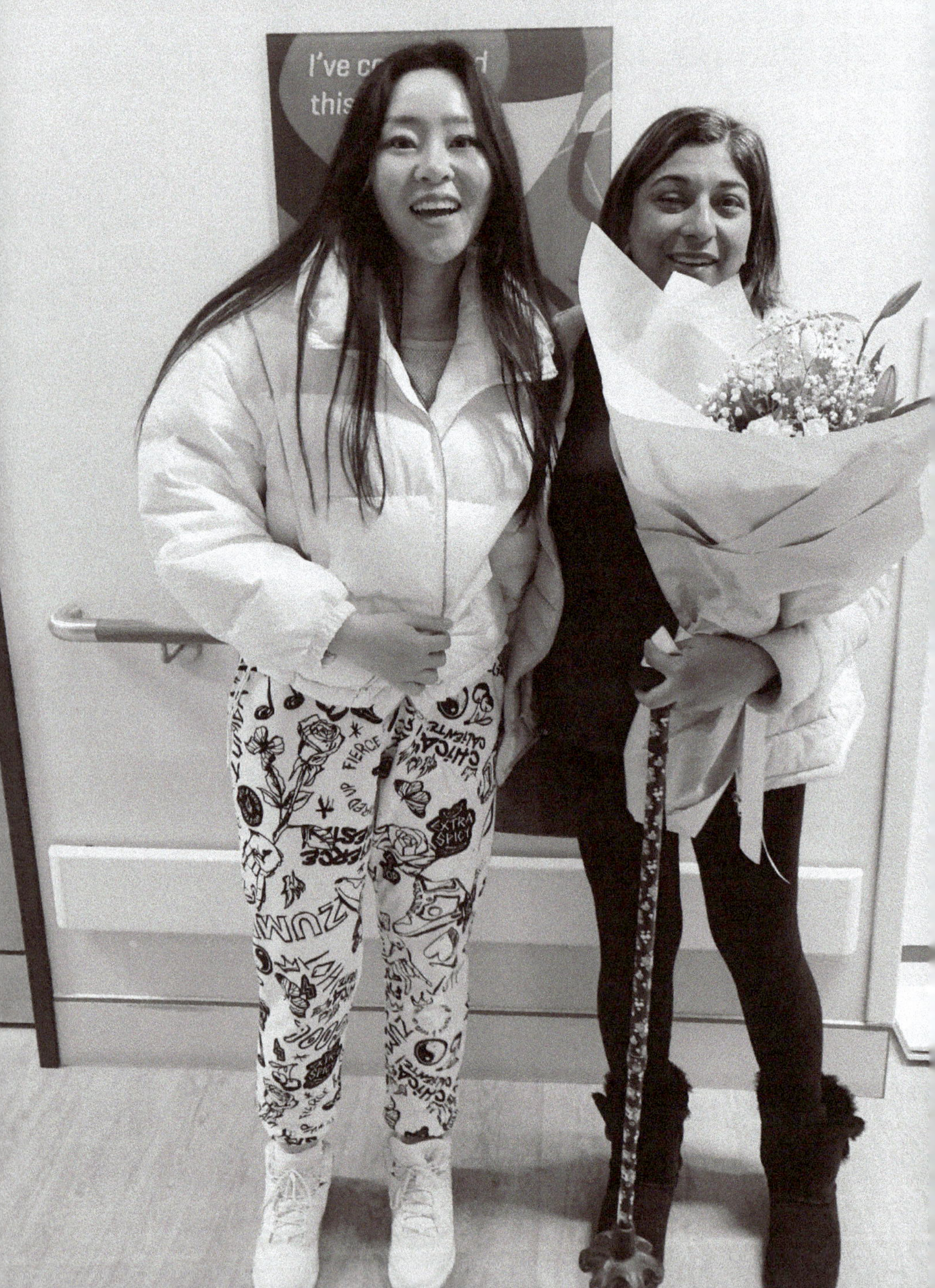

After radiation with Ariel